Why Do I Really Need Herbs?

What everyone should know about how
to get well, and stay well, with herbs.

by
Lorrie Medford, C.N.

LDN Publishing
P.O. Box 54007
Tulsa, Oklahoma 74155

WHY DO I REALLY NEED HERBS?
What everyone should know about how to get well, and stay well, with herbs.
ISBN #0-9676419-8-5
Copyright © 2004 Lorrie Medford, C.N.
LDN Publishing
P. O. Box 54007
Tulsa, OK 74155

Library of Congress Cataloging-in-Publishing Data

Medford, Lorrie, 1949

Why Do I Really Need Herbs?
Lorrie Medford, C.N.
International Standard Book Number: 0-9676419-8-5
1. Nutrition 2. Health 3. Herbal Supplements I.Title

NOTE: This book is not intended to take the place of medical advice. Readers are advised to consult their doctor or other qualified healthcare professional regarding treatment of their medical conditions.

Standard Process® is the exclusive distributor of MediHerb® in the United States. MediHerb and Standard Process are registered trademarks of MediHerb Pty. Ltd. and Standard Process Inc., respectively. MediHerb and Standard Process expressly disclaim any responsibility for and make no representations or warranties regarding any statement, information, materials, or content found on or included in this publication.

Printed in the United States of America

10 9 8 7 6 5 4 3 2 1 First U. S. Edition

(For ordering information, refer to the back pages of this book.)

The names of my clients have been changed. Any similarity to a real person is purely coincidental.

The fruit thereof shall be for meat,
and the leaf thereof for medicine.
Ezekiel 47:12

Contents

Foreword

There is a tremendous interest in the United States in the healing power of herbs. But along with this interest there is a great deal of confusion. Which expert do you listen to? There are some doctors and pharmacists who would have you believe that many popular herbs are dangerous, cause serious side effects or interact harmfully with conventional drugs. There are others who want you to believe that herbs have miraculous properties. There is also much confusion about important issues such as the quality of herbal products, the right dosage and which herbs to use for a particular health problem. So many times the poor consumer is misled and ends up taking an ineffective product for their health needs, or perhaps even worse, no herbs at all.

In this book Lorrie Medford provides an excellent introduction to many important issues such as the safe use of herbs, appropriate doses, key issues for herbal quality and the unique value of therapeutic plants. Throughout this book there is one important message: **that in most cases it is best to seek the advice of an expert who is trained in how to use herbs and understands the many complex issues.** In particular a suitably trained healthcare professional will be able to lead you to the right herbs at the right quality and in doses that will be effective.

I believe that herbs have a tremendous role to play in preventing and correcting a large number of health issues. This belief is based not just on my own clinical experience over 20 years, but also on the large amount of scientific research, including double-blind clinical trials, which has proven the efficacy of herbs in so many common health problems. In fact the benefits of herbs are often underestimated because of the ignorance of both the doctor and the patient. With this enlightening book by Lorrie Medford you can learn about the unique role and true value of therapeutic plants, especially when applied in a clinical setting.

Kerry Bone

Associate Professor

Australian College of Phytotherapy

Acknowledgements

Many thanks to professor and expert herbalist Kerry Bone, who so graciously reviewed my manuscript and wrote the foreword. I'm so grateful to you for your time and encouragement in writing this book. Thank you for dedicating your life to the science of herbal therapy and sharing it with the world in your classes and books.

Thanks also to herbalists Linda Ryan and Angela Hywood for being so willing to share your knowledge about the fascinating world of herbs. You are both superior herbalists and I'm grateful for your knowledge and support. Thanks for your encouragement to write this book as well.

Many thanks to my wonderful staff, Carolyn Clark, Anne Spears and Damon Harrison. You are always so willing to work on whatever project I have. Thanks for your ideas, suggestions and comments, and special thanks for your friendship and continual support.

Thanks also to Lori Oller for your great edit. Your comments always contribute greatly to my books and help the reader tremendously!

Thanks also to Lisa Simpson for your work on the cover. You are terrific and I appreciate your support.

Many thanks to my friend, Walter Scott for your support in producing this book. You have gone out of your way on several occasions and I am grateful.

Special thanks to my precious nephews, David and Kenath Johnson. David, I appreciate your ideas about humor for this book. You truly have a gift for writing! Kenath, thanks for all of your help with the index. You are so patient, careful, and so talented in working with computers. And special thanks to my twin sister, Jackie. Thanks for taking the time out of your busy schedule and four children, to review my manuscript. Your comments were great, and your English always was better than mine!

Many thanks to my precious clients who are always willing to take my nutrition and herbal suggestions to heart. Your testimonies will greatly help others.

And finally, again I thank God for life and purpose in Christ.

About the Author

Author and motivational speaker, Lorrie Medford has a BA in Communications and is a licensed Certified Nutritionist from The American Health Science University. She also holds certification as a personal trainer from ISSA (International Sports Science Association). She is a member of the Society of Certified Nutritionists, and is involved with the Oklahoma Speakers Association. Lorrie also serves on the Advisory Board for Standard Process, Inc.

In addition to writing this book, she has also written *Why Can't I Stay Motivated?*, *Why Can't I Lose Weight?*, *Why Can't I Lose Weight Cookbook*, *Why Do I Need Whole-Food Supplements?*, *Why Do I Feel So Lousy?*, *Why Am I So Wacky?*, *Why Am I So Grumpy, Dopey and Sleepy?* and *Why Eat Like Jesus Ate?*

A health researcher and journalist, Lorrie has studied nutrition, whole-foods cooking, herbs, health, fitness, and motivation for more than 30 years. Lorrie taught her weight-loss class at a local junior college and through her own business for more than 10 years, and has taught natural foods cooking classes in Spokane, Washington and Tulsa, Oklahoma for more than 5 years.

She shares her knowledge in her seminars, and through her thriving nutritional consultation practice, *Life Design Nutrition* in Tulsa, Oklahoma.

Lorrie has a rich history of community involvement teaching nutrition and is a sought-after speaker for civic groups, churches, hospitals, and wellness organizations.

She is uniquely qualified to write about health and fitness. Lorrie knows what it's like to be a *cranky calorie counter* obsessed with foods, dieting, and striving to be thin. After struggling with her weight for many years, Lorrie lost more than 35 pounds and has kept it off for more than twenty years.

Are You Confused About Herbs?

One way to get a glimpse of how a society spends their daily lives is to view their television commercials. Through American commercials, we can see that there are many people who probably suffer from pain, colds or the flu, and digestive problems. So if someone watched our television commercials, they might think that:

1. Americans have a lot of pain in their joints or muscles

2. Americans often are sick from colds or flu symptoms.

3. Americans have many types of digestive problems ranging from indigestion to constipation.

4. Americans need easier solutions for cleaning and washing their homes. (Oops! This is a good topic for another book, though!)

The idea of these commercials is that people just need to take this drug, or use this product and they will be happy-go-lucky and trouble free forever. Just take this drug for pain, and now you can dance all night. Just take this drug for the cold or flu symptoms, and you will never suffer again. Just take this drug for your digestive problems, and not only will the stomach pain leave, but you can continue to eat anything you want. And finally, just buy this kitchen or bathroom cleanser and you won't even have to get on the floor and scrub with your hands and knees. (Call me old fashioned, but I kind of like getting on my hands and knees to scrub the floor! But again...another book!)

The other day I was watching television when an advertisement caught my attention. An older, nice-looking couple was playing golf together, and gazing into each other's eyes as if they were newlyweds! Wondering what in the world they were advertising, I put down my papers and watched intently. In the background, music that I loved while I was growing up was being played. This well-made advertisement was like a mini-television show. Finally, at the end it was revealed that the product the commercial was promoting was medicine for diarrhea! Wow, it was hard to imagine which one was having the problem! But the solution was there: Take this drug.

However, the list of possible side effects from taking this drug was rattled off as though they were natural and innocuous. "Don't take this medicine if you have high-blood pressure, thyroid problems, and so on."

Hmmm, as the ad closed, I wondered if the manufacturer really believes that everyone knows whether they have high-blood pressure or not. Judging from my clients, many of them were not aware they had high-blood pressure until it was discovered at their last physical with their doctor.

As I thought more about the commercial, I remember thinking that there was never any mention about how they "got" the diarrhea. Maybe it's just me, but I've never wanted to take a drug unless I discovered why I needed it and more importantly, how I got the condition in the first place.

Later that night, there were more and more drug advertisements. Unlike Saturday morning, when all of the advertisements are for some type of gooey, sugary snack or food, in the evening there are literally dozens of advertisements for some type of drug.

Another advertisement that caught my attention featured various people who had words written with computer graphics across their stomachs with phrases like, "I feel bloated," or "I have gas."

Nearly every American over 35 has some type of stomach problem. And the answer again was, you guessed it—another drug!

Finally, the last commercial I saw was for a person with iron-deficiency anemia. Wow, a commercial that was advertising an iron supplement. Wonderful. The only problem was that it was a chemically made supplement for iron.

Your body can tell the difference between a natural mineral and a synthetic one. Here's a good example. My friend Hugh St. Onge told me about a woman who took a synthetic iron supplement and during an emergency surgery, they found 90 pharmaceutical iron tablets stuck in her colon!

More than likely, most people who are iron deficient are also deficient in hydrochloric acid, which helps break down minerals such as iron. People become deficient in hydrochloric acid if they eat too many refined sugars and carbohydrates. (You know, like candy, cake and ice cream!) But this commercial never mentioned food sources of iron, or hydrochloric acid. Through the years, I've helped hundreds if not thousands of people with iron deficiency anemia simply with whole-food supplements and dietary changes without any unnatural side effects such as constipation.

A few years ago, I wrote a book called *Why Do I Need Whole Food Supplements?* in which I explained how important it is that the vitamins we take be made from whole foods, and not synthetic chemicals. After thinking about these commercials, and how prevalent it is to take some type of drug for what ails you, I thought about the clients that I've helped with natural whole-food supplements and dietary changes. Most of them had dozens of questions about supplements and dietary suggestions they had heard over the years.

Being a health consumer is harder than ever. How do you know who to believe? Every day you see entertaining and wonderfully-produced commercials claiming the benefits of the latest and greatest medicinal drugs for whatever ails you. And besides, your mom and dad are taking these drugs and they, indeed, are not in pain.

Of course it has disturbed you that ever since taking these medications, your mom has high-blood pressure, dizzy spells and memory loss. You wonder about the medications she is taking. But her doctor says they are okay.

Before my mother passed away a few years ago, I remember having that discussion with her doctor, or should I say doctors. Everyone is specialized today. One doctor for the finger, one for the toe, nose, and so on!

But do these doctors talk to each other? Did my mother remember to tell doctor number one that she was taking a medication recommended by doctor number two? Well, one of the side effects of a certain drug that my mother was taking was unfortunately, loss of memory!

In reviewing mom's medications, I did notice, that she was finally taking a vitamin E supplement, for which I was surprised, having encouraged her again and again to take supplements. When I asked her about it, she simply replied, "Well, my heart doctor recommended it, along with fruits and vegetables." She was kind enough to add yes, she knew it was something I wanted (begged!) her to do years earlier, but now that the doctor told her she was motivated to do it.

Years ago, most doctors didn't believe supplements were important, but today many doctors do. Isn't it sometimes hard being a consumer? "Experts" have been contradicting each other for years. Today we have the internet. Now we can download more contradictory information—only faster!

Who should take care of your health? Who should have all of the answers? We are trained in this country and other industrialized countries to look to doctors for advice.

After all, look again at the television commercials. Do you have a headache? Here is a quick fix, take this drug. It's not like there are other options on television. There is not a commercial following the first commercial saying, "Hey, would you like an alternative to a medicine for your headache? What about taking white willow bark, or some other herbal supplement for pain?" When was the last time you saw an advertisement like that?

Does anyone wonder "why" they got the headache in the first place? I had a female client who complained of headaches for years. I made several dietary and supplement suggestions which literally changed her entire health profile and even her life. We found the cause of the problem which, in her case, was a severe deficiency of the B complex vitamins. She no longer needed to take a drug to handle the symptoms.

If You Feel Confused, You Are Not Alone

Most of my clients come in with a bag or two of vitamins and medications that they have been taking. I'm still surprised when they pull out one, two, three, four, five, six, seven and even more medications!

If they have come to me with a weight or energy problem, and they are taking these medications, their weight gain is not a big mystery. All of these medications influence a person's energy and metabolism.

These side effects happen for a reason.

I often think about a female client named Janice who came to see me years ago. I will never forget how she cried during the entire first appointment. I found literally a dozen vitamin/mineral deficiencies and imbalances in her body and reported them to her as the appointment progressed. I will never forget what she told me at the end of the appointment either. "If you didn't have any answers for me, I was going to kill myself after this appointment!" Well, thank God I had lots of answers! Janice reported that the crying stopped about three days later, and she sent me a lovely bouquet of flowers to thank me. She was back to work within a couple of months, after having been unable to work for quite a long time.

I was so excited that I could help Janice and people like her. You see, I discovered that Janice had been prescribed six different antidepressants, apparently from different doctors. The thing was, she didn't have an antidepressant deficiency. She had numerous vitamin and mineral deficiencies, though.

Three Important Questions

I wrote this book especially for people who have been told they need medications for some health problem **for the rest of their lives.** Unfortunately, they don't want to continue taking these medications if they produced:

1. No results.
2. Only temporary symptom relief.
3. Side effects that cause even more health problems, such as weight gain or headaches.

Most of these people are looking for natural and safe solutions to their health problems. They would like to try herbs, but wonder...

1. Are there really natural herbal alternatives to the medications I am taking?
2. Are herbs safe? Will they interact with drugs?
3. How do you know which herbs to buy? How do you read the label? How do you know the right amount to take?

Where Do You Need Help?

Most people don't have the time to thoroughly investigate the medications they are taking or get the right information to learn about herbs and possible herb/drug interactions. So when they watch the television news report about the possible dangers of an herb, they just stop taking it.

But most people have heard at one time or another about an herb that worked! And for all of the cautions about taking herbal supplements, I doubt that most people know that nearly 150,000 to 200,000 people die from properly prescribed medications yearly. In the past thirty years, I've only heard of a handful of deaths linked to herbs, and even these were questionable due to the medications that were taken along with the herb. (If they were taking an herb along with a medication, isn't it a bit unfair to blame everything on the herb, which has few side effects, and not on the drugs, which often can result in many side effects?)

In this book, I'll tell you why you should consider taking herbal supplements, why all herbal supplements on the market aren't the same, and how to safely take herbs. Here's a review of the three parts of this book and their chapters.

Part One: Why Take Herbs?

Chapter 1 Defines real health.

Chapter 2 Looks at the history of how humans have gotten well through the past centuries and who decided how we get well in America.

Chapter 3 Defines herbs and gives several reasons to take herbal supplements.

Chapter 4 Compares herbs to drugs.

Chapter 5 Gives more information about drugs, how they work, and the side effects of drugs.

Part Two: How to Buy and Take Herbs

Chapter 6 Explains the difference between various types of herbal supplements and how to read an herbal label.

Chapter 7 Answers the important question about the safety of herbs.

Chapter 8 Gives you tips on how to take herbs.

Part Three: Herbs for Life

Chapter 9 Lists popular herbs for great health.

Chapter 10 Gives you several handy herbal recipes.

Chapter 11 Tells you how to find great herbs and a natural health professional.

Okay, let's go to Part One which addresses the question of why we should even consider taking herbs.

PART ONE

Why Take Herbs?

Chapter One

What Is Real Health?

Are you "healthy," except for headaches, earaches, allergies, toothaches, bladder infections, and so on?

Clients often surprise me when they begin to discuss their health history. For example, a client named Erma recently came in requesting help for weight loss. When we finished discussing our strategy for weight loss, she finally mentioned that she had allergies. Since she waited until the end of the appointment to address this, I thought perhaps it was not very significant. I was shocked when she said that she had severe allergies her entire life! When I asked why she waited until the end to tell me about it, she told me that she didn't expect that there was anything I could do for her. Besides, her medications helped, and she was told that she would just have to live with them. Otherwise, she was "healthy." I'm glad she told me because one of the side effects of the allergy medication she was taking was weight gain. Fortunately, I was able to help her lose weight and eliminate allergy symptoms naturally.

Are we really "healthy"?

Think about our health statistics. Today, the top three killers include heart disease, cancer and diabetes.

Heart disease has been the leading cause of death in our country for years. In fact, over a million people die yearly from heart disease.

According to the author of *Prescription Alternatives,* the American Heart Association estimated that the cost of cardiovascular disease as far back as 1994 alone was $128 billion dollars![1] The medical care costs for Americans with chronic diseases such as these total more than $400 billion annually.

According to the American Cancer Society, one in three Americans are expected to get cancer in their lifetime. The National Institutes of Health estimates that cancer costs Americans $60.9 billion a year in medical bills.[2] The World Health Organization (WHO) estimates deaths from cancer will double over the next 20 years.[3]

The Surgeon General's Report of 2001 warned that soon obesity may overtake the previous number of deaths from smoking. According to Surgeon General Dr. David Satcher, nearly 65% of Americans are overweight, and 13% of our children are overweight. Approximately 300,000 deaths a year are associated with overweight and obesity.[4] In spite of all of our technology, drugs, and new and improved foods, supplements and fitness equipment, we have now become the fattest nation on the planet!

Uh-oh! This isn't good health!

What Is Our Standard Of Health?

How many people do you know who really feel good every day and are not dealing with some type of health problem? People today don't really know what it's like to really be healthy or feel good! But who defined health for us?

If people were well with our current model of health care, I wouldn't even be writing this book. But they aren't. They are sick. They are tired. They are overweight. And for all the money they spend on doctors and drugs, our health statistics are not improving! **We have the most sophisticated technologically advanced healthcare system yet we are one of the sickest countries in the new world.**

I think it's because we don't even know what health is anymore.

The World Health Organization has a great definition of health: "A state of complete physical, mental, and social well-being and not merely the absence of disease or infirmity." This definition was written in 1948![5]

Most of us never really experience times of "complete physical well-being." For example, every day I ask people about their daily bowel movements. I had to revise the question early on in my practice when I realized that for some people, their definition of "being regular" was once a week! If you've read any of my previous books, you'll know that being "regular" should mean at least once or twice a day!

We were designed to live long, healthy lives. If we're not healthy, somewhere along the way we have interfered with this process. We accept common symptoms of headaches or allergies as "normal" because everyone our age has them. But they are not normal—any more than it's normal for small children and teenagers to get arthritis and heart disease. One hundred years ago this was unheard of. Why is it "normal" now? It's not normal; it's just **common** now because children and teens are not getting as much nutrition as their grandparents did.

What About Our Grandparents?

For years, I've heard people justify smoking, drinking and their poor eating habits because their grandfather drank, smoke, or ate poorly and after all, he lived to be 90.

But guess what? Today, people who smoke, drink and eat poorly are not living to be 90! In fact, they are dying in their 40s, 50s and 60s!

Things have changed! In the early 18th century and prior, people were healthier. They lived on farms and worked hard. They ate whole foods and more fruits and vegetables. They ate kale, beets and broccoli. (Today, if I suggest a client eats kale, beets or broccoli, they might either ask what they are, or run out of my office!) In the past, if someone got cancer, they lived a fairly long, healthy life in spite of it! They didn't die from cancer. Since drugs were not easily available, herbs and folk medicine were commonly used.

Cancer expert Dr. Patrick Quillin, in his book, *Beating Cancer With Nutrition,* believes that at least 40% of cancer patients will die from malnutrition, not the cancer itself.[6]

Did you know that fifty years ago, the big killer diseases were smallpox, diphtheria and tuberculosis? These illnesses were caused by infectious bacteria. Did you know there was no reported incidence of heart disease until the early 1900s? Just one hundred years ago, only 3% of Americans died from cancer.

It may surprise you to know that in the early 19th century, doctors looked at your hair, skin and nails, and inquired about your lifestyle to determine the cause of health problems. Often they were aware of subclinical nutritional deficiencies.

For example, pale skin color was and still is linked to B12 deficiency, iron-deficiency anemia, adrenal insufficiency or hypothyroidism. Skin problems such as acne did and still does indicate zinc and vitamin A deficiencies. These doctors recommended foods, supplements and herbs for health.

Today, people have no idea of the nutritional deficiencies they might have. Some clients have left my office with a dosage sheet which listed 18-20 nutrients they were deficient in. (On a good day, most people lack at least 7 or 8!)

Today, most people's diets aren't good, so their immune systems are weaker than their grandparents were. When they get sick, they have to work doubly hard to overcome diseases such as heart disease and cancers.

Symptoms of a Weakened Immune System

I don't think people realize that disease doesn't necessarily happen in a month, or a year. Disease comes from nutritional deficiencies and poor living habits over years and years.

I explained what I consider the four stages of disease in one of my previous books, entitled, *Why Do I Feel So Lousy?*[7]:

1. Poor digestion
2. A sluggish liver
3. Poor elimination
4. A weakened immune system

When the immune system is weakened, this eventually leads to further degeneration and disease. You can become susceptible to every bacteria or virus that comes around. You get headaches. You get arthritis. You feel pain. That will get your attention!

Take a look at some symptoms of a weakened immune system.

Check the following if it applies to you:

1. Do you have brain fog?
2. Do you have watery, itchy eyes?
3. Do you have aches or pains in your joints?
4. Do you have a chronic cough or sinus problems?
5. Do you have shortness of breath or asthma?
6. Do you have allergies?
7. Do you have constipation or diarrhea?
8. Do you experience hot flashes or an overheating of the body?
9. Do you feel groggy upon awakening?
10. Do you frequently have headaches?
11. Do you have root canals or mercury amalgam fillings?
12. Do you have bags or circles under your eyes?
13. Do you frequently feel depressed or experience low energy levels?
14. Do you suffer from frequent infections or chemical sensitivities?

Did you answer yes to any of these questions? Most of us live without ever considering these stages of degeneration. Most of us don't even know why we get a stomachache or any other pain for that matter! But living with any of these symptoms is not health!

The Most Important Factor

Heart disease, cancer, diabetes and a weakened immune system are "lifestyle" diseases. For the past twenty years, a tremendous amount of research has proved that malnutrition is a major contributor to disease and that proper nutrition can help **prevent** disease. **Now we know that many of these deaths could have been prevented with proper nutrition and lifestyle!**

Foods that our grandparents ate such as kale, broccoli, and beets, for example, have phytochemical compounds that boost the production of anti-cancer enzymes within hours of being eaten. (Too bad they don't taste like pizza!) We now know that if we want to be healthy, we have to eat foods that are designed for our bodies.

But did you know that throughout the centuries, herbs, along with food, played a large part in getting and keeping people well? Herbs are beneficial for so many reasons. Not only do they support the healing process naturally, but they also contain nutrition that is often lacking in today's modern, processed foods.

So now you might be wondering, if herbs helped, why haven't we heard more about them before now? Why do we take so many drugs instead?

If you are unhealthy, overweight, or dealing with some type of disease, it's probably not entirely your fault! Think about who taught you to eat. Who defined health for you? When were you taught that you can prevent disease? And who taught you to take drugs?

Let's take a short look at who really decided how we should get well.

Chapter Two

Who Decided How We Get Well?

Who decided how we should get well throughout the past centuries? Perhaps prehistoric cavemen watched their pet dinosaur, Fido, eat grass when he got sick. Fido recovered, so they decided that grass must be okay to eat when you get sick!

They probably tasted herbs and grasses, and they might have said, "Ummm, this one tastes good! Or, "This one helps me sleep," and so on. (I pity the poor Neanderthal who first sampled the laxative-type herb Cascara!)

It's not like there were 24 hour herbal drug stores on every corner of the street; they were lucky to even get food to eat back then!

What happened that we went from living to age ninety and symptom-free to dying of heart disease and cancer in our 50s and 60s? When was the shift made from simple, home remedies to pharmaceutical drugs? And why haven't we been educated about what health really is and how to prevent disease? Whose fault is it?

In order to fully understand this shift, we need to look at American history regarding our food, farming and advertising.

Following World War I, Americans moved from the country to the city. According to Mark Anderson, in his well-researched book, *Empty Harvest,* government food and drug regulation served the long-shelf life demands of food processors (regardless of nutritional quality). After generations of Americans eating whole, unprocessed foods, science showed the food industry easier ways to make quick profits. Processing methods included foods that were now bleached, refined, chemically preserved, pasteurized, sterilized, homogenized, hydrogenated, artificially colored, highly sugared, highly salted, synthetically fortified, canned, and generally exposed to hundreds of new man-made chemicals.[8]

Mark explains how Dr. Royal Lee, a pioneer in the field of nutrition (considered by some to be one of the world's greatest nutritionists) and other health pioneers tried to expose the truth that diseases such as dental caries and diabetes were caused by sugar and processed foods. Unfortunately, Dr. Lee was branded a "racketeer" because he promoted whole, natural, unadulterated foods with their vitamins and minerals intact. Mark said, "The tragedy of my parents' generation is that they grew up listening to Betty Crocker instead of Royal Lee. Sadly, his work was condemned as dangerous to the public. So while Camel cigarettes and sugar were left to reap their profits, federal judges told Dr. Lee to stifle his writings and lectures, or go to jail."[9] We now know for certain that dietary deficiencies caused by sugar lead to degenerative and infectious diseases.

In several of my books, I've mentioned that the Food Guide Pyramid hasn't always been the standard that the government promoted in our country. There have been several government-recommended dietary standards throughout the years. A look at the food pyramids of other nations reveal not only more balanced nutrition, but a focus on healthier foods. (See my book, *Why Eat Like Jesus Ate?* for more details.) None of the American standards were tested ahead of time to see how they would work. (Most panel "experts" who design these pyramids are linked to the processed food industry.[10]) We now know that because of the high carbohydrate intake of the Food Guide Pyramid, two-thirds of Americans are overweight!

You'll often hear drug commercials say, "When exercise and a change in diet don't work to lower your cholesterol, take this drug." What "diet" are they referring to? If it's the standard American one, be careful!

America is an affluent society, blessed with not only natural foods, but highly processed foods. In the last ten years, more than ten thousand "convenient (processed) foods" have been introduced in the United States. Most people eat more than 200 grams of processed carbohydrates every day. Where do we get them and who is telling us to eat them?

How To Get Fat

The largest manufacturing industry in America is the processed food industry. In a television special in 2003, Peter Jennings did a report entitled, "How to Get Fat Without Really Trying." He said that in the 1930s the government began to subsidize farmers to save them from financial ruin; the problem is that they never stopped.[11]

In this report, Jennings showed what the food pyramid would look like if it reflected where government subsidies went. Sugars and fats (which are at the top of the pyramid and should be eaten sparingly) receive twenty times more government subsidies than fruits and vegetables.

Something that most Americans don't know is that the most heavily subsidized crop in America is corn. We think of corn as the sweet corn that we eat at picnics. But subsidized corn is everywhere—it's the cheap raw material for the giant food industry. This corn is fed to chicken and cattle to make them grow fatter, faster (which holds down the cost of meat.) Corn makes people fatter, too!

This corn is processed and put in thousands of high-calorie processed foods that Americans eat every day—from pop corn, processed vegetable corn oil, candy, pretzels and hot dogs to high-fructose corn syrup. Jennings says that Americans eat more than **three times the amount of corn in the form of sweeteners** than any other form. Through these farm subsidies, the government controls the way food is grown and processed in this country. Yet when asked if there was a connection between the obesity epidemic and the food industry, the spokesperson replied that people should make the right choices!

Never mind that the government allows thousands of products to be introduced each year; ninety percent of which are packaged junk foods we should eat less of. Paul Stitt, an author who spent years as a food scientist for two of the country's top food industry corporations calls the manufacturers of processed foods, "Food Giants."

In his eye-opening book, *Beating the Food Giants,* Stitt talks about the casualties of processed food addiction which he calls "Can't Eat Just One Syndrome." What causes this syndrome and what's it doing to our bodies? Paul explains that "Food Giants" know if they add enough fat, sugar and salt, Americans will eat almost anything.[12]

> Have you ever eaten just one Oreo cookie? Bet you can't either. They look so sweet and innocent! What you should realize is that the Nabisco Company spent millions developing that formula so that you can't eat just one. It contains 23 different appetite stimulants... I saw the recipe and I was aghast. It's not easy to make a cookie that will hook every last American![13]

And you thought it was all because of your lack of willpower!

In her book, *Food Politics,* Marion Nestle reports that the food industry spends $33 billion dollars a year to promote these foods.[14]

Additionally, more than $12 billion dollars are spent yearly to promote foods to kids.[15] Most of these foods are highly processed foods, turning candy into breakfast cereals. Is it any wonder that now 13-14% of our children are overweight?

How Did This Happen?

The American Dietetic Association (ADA) which has more than 65,000 members, provides public education and sets nutritional guidelines for hospitals and schools. The

ADA also receives substantial contributions from groups such as the National Livestock and Meat Board, Sugar Association, and from companies such as McDonald's, Coca-Cola, and other snack food companies.[16]

A *New York Times* article written by Marian Burros explains that the (ADA) takes the "wishy-washy stance" that there are not "good or bad foods," because the ADA relies on food industry money. This means they would never criticize the food industry.[17] If there aren't any "bad" foods, why are we so sick and tired? We can't rely on "traditional, governmental" sources for our nutritional information when these sources are linked to the marketing of processed foods.

Since the main education comes from governmental publications, it looks like our government has done a great job of making us fat, sick and tired! Everywhere we go, we have access to food, from vending machines in gas stations to snacks in laundromats.

The government recommends we Americans eat nine servings of fresh fruits and vegetables daily. However, our government also encourages the sale of sugary foods and sodas in vending machines in schools. Sugar depresses their immune systems and make it hard for children to concentrate!

Contrast that with countries like Russia, where it has been common to give their children a drink called kefir when they get to school. Kefir has been known for years to be an incredible super food which builds a strong immune system.

When Did Drugs Enter the Scene?

Have you ever wondered how pharmaceutical drugs became so popular?

In the 1930s, people were powerfully persuaded to smoke cigarettes because of advertising campaigns. People thought if it was advertised, it was the truth. In his book, Mark Anderson reprinted a Camel cigarette ad from 1937 that said that Camels helped people digest their food![18] Advertising creates trends and influences cultures. People later discovered that cigarettes caused emphysema and lung cancer and they were finally taken off television (not off the shelf!)

Drugs are relatively new kids on the block. It's funny how when something is frequently on television, like advertisements for drugs, people assume they must be okay. Or, if they are being advertised, they must be the best way for us to get well. When I grew up, there were few drug advertisements on television. Perhaps there was an advertisement for headache or cold remedies here and there. Today, advertisements for drugs are as popular as common household cleaners.

The shift to drugs as our final answer began at the dawn of the 19th century when people moved from farms to the cities. TV dinners replaced home-cooked meals. People saw drugs as more of a quick fix than herbs were. Eventually, simple folk remedies and herbal formulas fell by the wayside. As large food industries overtook the grocery industry, drug companies now overtook the herbal industry.

Did you know that most of the drugs that people are taking today were only developed in the last 50 or 60 years? The average person over 60 who comes into my office is on between 7 to 10 medications. Yet their grandparents may not have taken any medications. Let's hit the highlights of the history of herbs and drugs.

The First Healing Agents

Every culture has herbal roots and traditions since herbs have been around since the beginnings of civilization. Written accounts of herbal medicines are found throughout the world since nearly every primitive culture discovered the healing properties of herbs that grew in their environment.

Most herbs were discovered through experimenting or by trial and error. As they learned about the type of plant and the results they got, that was the very beginning of herbal medicine as we know it today!

Even ancient scriptures say that herbs were always a part of God's plan for healing man. Genesis 3:18 says, "And thou shalt eat the herb of the field." In Ezekiel 47:12, Ezekiel said that the "leaves of the tree" were for man's healing. Rev. 22:2 says, "And the leaves of the tree were for the healing of the nations."

Herbs Have Been Used for Centuries

Most of the history of healing has been done with herbs. Not for one year, but for thousands of years. Not for one century, but for a dozen or more centuries. **Herbs were, and still are, the major agents our bodies were designed to use.**

Even today, the World Health Organization reports that 80% of the world's population uses herbs and foods as their primary healing agents.[19]

Our current medical system is only about a few hundred years old. **The more research I've done, the more I've wondered how in the world we ever stopped using herbs as our primary healing agents.** Think about this. Plants have always been the basis of healing agents since the earliest days. The same herbs that are around today have been around for thousands of years! So what happened?

Early History of Herbs

Ancient Chinese and Egyptian writings both indicate the use of herbs as medicines as far back as 4,000 years B.C. The Egyptians wrote about herbs and were known to use garlic, mint, senna, flaxseed, celery and onions.

Hippocrates (460-367 B.C.) was known as the "Father of Modern Medicine." As far as we know he was the first man who practiced medicine promoting the use of herbs and practicing a system of medicine which focused on treating the person rather than the symptoms of disease.

Everyone has probably heard the condensed version of the Hippocratic oath which some physicians take when they enter their practice. It basically said, "I won't give deadly medicines to anyone or otherwise harm them." I came across the Hippocratic oath in the classic edition of a book written by Jethro Kloss called *Back to Eden*. It was first published in 1939, and it has been reprinted most every year since.

Here is the oath: "I will follow that system of regimen which, according to my ability and judgment, I consider for the benefit of my patients, and abstain from whatever is deleterious and mischievous. I will give no deadly medicine to anyone if asked, nor suggest any such counsel."[20]

What you might not know is that Hippocrates believed in natural healing. He never advocated drug therapy; he was one of our first "natural" (naturopathic) docs! An interesting addendum in Jethro Kloss' book, "...nature could heal the body and that the physician was only nature's helper." Hippocrates treated his patients with herbs, proper diet, fresh air, and exercise. He mentioned 400 herbs in his writings, one-third of which are still in use.[21]

Many people and cultures kept the history of herbal medicines alive. According to Kloss, Avicenna was an Arab herbalist who lived in the 11th century and traveled widely, cataloging the use of herbs as medicine. He wrote 100 books and eventually wrote a standard in Europe and Asia for medical education based on herbs, called *Canon of Medicine.* Avicenna believed that there was a plant that could cure every ailment.[22] Was he an optimist or just a great herbalist?

Australian herbal expert and author, Kerry Bone, in his textbook, *Principles and Practice of Phytotherapy,* reports that a Greek physician named Dioscorides collected information on 500 plants and remedies in the first century AD and recorded one of the foundational herbal books entitled *Materia Medica.*[23] Dioscorides is credited for classifying herbs according to how they work in the body.

England Herbals

Following the invention of the printing press in the 15th century, hundreds of herbal books were printed. The 15th, 16th and 17th centuries were great ages of herbals in England according to herbalist Michael Castleman.[24]

In 1653, an English physician named Nicholas Culpeper wrote *The Complete Herbal and English Physician,* one of the first respected herbals that the lay person could use. His book has been reprinted through countless editions to the present day.

He was a controversial physician, loved by the people and ridiculed by the doctors. While his work was criticized by the medical establishment of the day, apothecaries, midwives and common people respected him for giving them access to professional, herbal, medical information.[25]

Early American Medicine

Bone reports that our modern herbology is derived from European herbology. Immigrants from Europe were the first to bring European herbal plants here. In the early 19th century, the majority of immigrants to North America were Europeans. Since they lived hundreds of miles from doctors, they had to rediscover their self-sufficiency in health combining their (imported) old European home remedies with native North American and Indian remedies as well. Their experience provided the rediscovery of traditional herbal medicine.[26] The combination of European herbology and knowledge of herbs from the native American Indians led to American folk medicine.[27]

Medical practice at that time included such outdated and dangerous remedies as the use of mercury, violent laxatives and "bleeding" people, all three of which could kill them![28]

According to Bone, one of early America's leading herbalists was Samuel Thomson, known as the "white Indian doctor," who was introduced to herbs by a midwife versed in Indian herbology. Thomson was horrified by the medical remedies used of the day. The book in which he propagated his views was a runaway publishing success across the East and Mid West at the time.[29] Another group who inspired the use of herbs at that time were the "Eclectics" who were

America's first scientific herbalists. They adopted the name "eclectic" to describe their herb-based approach, which combined European, Asian, and Indian herbalism.[30] Kerry Bone told me that some of our best herbs such as Golden Seal and Echinacea were popularized by the Eclectics after they learned about them from the Native Americans. The Eclectic legacy lives on in herbal medicine programs at the nation's top two naturopathic medical schools, the National College of Naturopathic Medicine in Portland, Oregon and John Bastyr University in Seattle, Washington.[31]

Most people don't know that naturopathy was popular in the U.S. in the 19th century. Naturopathy relies on herbal remedies combined with fasting, exercise, fresh air, sunshine, diet and water to help the body to heal itself. At that time there were many naturopathic doctors (N.D.).

According to Jethro Kloss, the introduction of naturopathy in America was probably attributed to Samuel Thomson. Along with herbs, he used sweat baths, diet and massage. His motto was "To make every man his own physician."[32]

Bone explains that the main colleges of Thomsonism, along with those of homeopathy were 'invited' to come within the umbrella of established medical training in discussions held with the American Medical Association at the turn of the century. He calls it an example of the establishment trying to eliminate "radicals" by accommodating them.[33]

W. H. Cook was another doctor who attempted to link the discoveries of medical science to herbal-based traditional approaches. Cook believed that ideal medicine should support the recuperative functions of the body. Unfortunately, this practice died down and entire schools were moved to England. Bone reports:[34]

> Thomsonism traveled to Britain...Their approaches formed the foundation of the oldest body of medical herbalism in the Western world, the National Institute of Medical Herbalists,

established in 1864. Although the vigour of the American pioneers faded in the following century, their ideas at least survived on foreign shores while they singularly failed to do so after the AMA takeover at home.

In the late 1800s, Western medicine evolved, and the use of herbs, which for most of history had been mainstream, began to be considered "unscientific" and fell into obscurity.

The American Medical Association

After the change of the century, the onslaught of the American Medical Association led to the decline and disappearance of Eclectic medicine. The last school of Eclectic medicine closed in 1939.

In the early 1900s herbal remedies were widely used until drug companies began isolating these compounds and making drugs. The old herbals have been replaced by the Physician's Desk Reference, an extensive listing of pharmaceutical drugs which includes contraindications and possible side effects.

The medical system became "allopathic," which refers to the general practice of medicine today which uses drug therapy. Eventually, allopathic medicine took hold and Americans have become conditioned to take drugs for instant relief.

Even as late as 1960, some herbs were still listed in the Physician's Desk Reference. Unfortunately, drugs began to evolve and have replaced wonderful herbal medicines that had been used for centuries. **It only took some fifty years to snuff out the tradition of herbs that were used for centuries!**

Herbalism Today

The herbalists in Great Britain, called Medical Herbalists, are the successors of Hippocrates. England is far ahead of the U.S. in this respect; naturopathic doctors still have permission to practice in England and even English royalty use herbal doctors.

Herbs such as Echinacea and St. John's Wort are commonly used by medical doctors in Europe. Phytomedicines are recognized in Europe where they are categorized as "plant-derived" drugs. In Germany, phytomedicines are considered ethical drugs and they are commonly prescribed by physicians and dispensed by pharmacists.

Even in the more modern areas of Europe, herbal remedies are considered either front-line or complements to drugs that mainstream medicine offers. In Germany nearly 700 plant based remedies are available and 70% of physicians prescribe them. The Commission E has supported the wider acceptance of herbs in Germany. Commission E is a group of physicians, pharmacologists and scientists appointed by the German Federal Health Agency. They report the most commonly used herbs giving information on dosing and possible side effects.[35]

So now you might wonder why American doctors don't know more about herbs? By and large, physicians have looked down on folk medicine and like most doctors of the past, view herbal medicines as primitive and backward. Many American physicians not only don't prescribe herbal supplements, they actively speak out against them.

American doctors' knowledge of herbs involves what they read in medical journal articles, which often focus on the dangers of using herbs irresponsibly. Compare that to the early 1900s, when medical doctors used herbology and even took herbal courses as part of medical school training. Yet today medical schools ignore the history of the traditional use of herbs. **Most doctors don't know that until the 20th century, most medicines were herbal.**[36]

It's certainly about time that we returned to our true roots of the use of herbs and natural health care.

Let's move on to Chapter Three which gives you great reasons why we should take herbs.

What Are Herbs and Why Should I Take Them?

Maybe you don't really understand what herbs are, and you only have a vague idea of where they come from and how to get them. I think for many people, their idea of an herbalist is someone who lives in the country, has a long beard, frequently eats garlic, and has no real friends!

So what are herbs? They're simply plants. In the technical sense, herbs are plants which have medicinal value. Their medicinal value could come from the leaves, flowers, stems, berries, seeds, bark or roots of plants.

When people ask me about herbs, they find it interesting when I tell them they are probably taking them already. I often ask them, "Do you ever eat at Italian, Indian or Mexican restaurants?" If you do, you've eaten garlic, basil, cayenne pepper, cumin, tumeric and curry powder. They're all herbs, but beside their medicinal value, they also make great flavoring for foods.

Today, the Chinese are the foremost herbalists. They have drawn on thousands of years of experience in identifying and using herbs, used as a preventative first and then as necessary, a cure. Herbs found their way into Chinese kitchens as well.

Centuries ago, Hippocrates referred to the healing power of herbs when he wrote the popular sentence: "Let your food be your medicine and let your medicine be your food."

Think about a common food such as garlic. Known as a popular spice, it's also an herb and a medicine. Garlic has been studied perhaps more than any one single herb. It's medicinal benefits include lowering blood pressure, lowering cholesterol levels and use as an anti-bacterial. Garlic is a great example of a food which is an incredible healing agent.

While we think of vegetable plants as food, and drugs as medicine, this isn't how the majority of people on the earth see it. As I mentioned in the last chapter, medicinal drugs in this country are fairly new. Plant foods have been here for thousands of years.

Why Haven't Americans Known About Herbs?

Most Americans have no idea of the long term historical use of herbs around the world. Why don't we know more about herbs? Here are some reasons.

1. We have never been taught about herbs in our educational system.

2. Most herbal formulas that people use have not been very effective. I've had clients bring in the supplements that they are taking and in the majority of cases, they bring several herbs such as Saw Palmetto or St. John's Wort that simply never worked. (In Chapter Six you'll see how not all herbal supplements are alike, and how you can get positive results with properly prepared herbs.)

3. Many people are afraid of herbs. There seems to be an unknown mystery about herbs. Perhaps they have heard about toxic or poisonous herbs. Perhaps they think of herbals as secretive, dangerous, or being brewed with mysterious agents involving religious cults, which is far from the truth.

4. Many people fear interactions with medicinal drugs. Since most people know about drugs, they may fear interactions with the drugs they are taking, which is a legitimate fear. (I address this in Chapter Seven.)

5. Often people see herbs as primitive and backward in view of our high-tech culture.

6. But by far the main reason that people don't know about herbs is that their primary health care provider is a

doctor, not an herbalist. Most doctors use drugs, not herbs. So most Americans aren't exposed to herbs. Where does everyone hear about drugs? Television commercials are used to "program" the American public! Yet almost everything you hear about health on television is financially or politically motivated.

And most people have not been encouraged to know their own bodies. There seems to be a "the least you know, the better" mentality in the doctor's office.

However, things are changing. The 1994 Dietary Supplement and Health and Education Act (DSHEA) lifted decades of barriers that made it difficult to bring supplements to market. This act made it easier for manufacturers to make general, not specific health claims for products as long as they had scientific backing. For example, they can write that a particular supplement "supports joint health" rather than "cures arthritis." This act has made the practice of herbal medicine more popular. Today nearly 50 million Americans use herbal supplements.

How Do Herbs Work?

Herbs used in herbal medicine are also known as "botanical medicine" or, in Europe as "phytotherapy" or "phytomedicine." Today's current herbal knowledge combines the best of ancient, historical writings and medical science to understand what makes herbs work.

There are a few basic types of herbs: nutritive or food herbs and medicinal herbs.

Nutritive or food herbs offer the body nutrients that it doesn't receive either because of environmental deficiencies in the soil, or a poor diet. As concentrated sources of nutrients, food herbs add nutritional value to your diet. Examples are: garlic, barley grass, bee pollen, bilberry, rosehips, and broccoli.

Medicinal herbs really act to balance the body, with positive effect on tissues, organs and glands. Medicinal herbs include a variety of types of herbs which are often categorized by their "action" on our physiology.

The component of the plant that actually heals an organ or tissue is called the "active" compound or chemical. What these herbal "actions" do is describe the way the remedy affects our bodies. A good example is the flavone glycosides found in ginkgo which are the natural chemicals that support better circulation. That's why ginkgo is commonly recommended for people with circulatory or memory problems.

Plants may contain hundreds of these active components.

Knowing the actions of a plant is vital. For example, you wouldn't want to give an herb that makes a person feel calm to someone who needed to be alert!

There are nearly a hundred "actions" or descriptions of the properties of herbs. When I attended an herbal seminar, so many unfamiliar words were rolling off the herbalist's tongue that for a moment I thought I was in a foreign language class! Some examples are: diaphoretic, emmenagogue, anthelmintic and emetic. Let me give you just a few examples (easy ones that I could pronounce!) that you might be familiar with.

Adaptogenic These herbs increase our resistance to stress by supporting the adrenal glands.

Antibiotic These herbs help the body's immune system to destroy the growth of micro-organisms.

Anti-fungal These herbs act against and destroy fungi.

Anti-inflammatory These herbs help to reduce inflammation in the body.

Antiviral These herbs destroy viruses in the body.

Demulcent These herbs soothe and protect the mucous membranes in the body.

Diuretic These herbs increase the flow of urine to relieve water retention.

Hepatic These herbs tone and strengthen the liver and can increase the flow of bile.

Nervine These herbs strengthen and restore the nervous system.

Sedative These herbs are used to relieve irritability.

Vasoconstrictor These herbs help to constrict blood vessels and raise blood pressure.

Vasodilator These are herbs that expand blood vessels and lower blood pressure.

The list could go on and on; I've just given you a handful so you can see how versatile and beneficial herbs are. You would have to consult an herbal textbook to study all of these actions. But you can see how vital it is that you would know the action of an herb. For example, if you wanted to raise someone's blood pressure, you would use a vasoconstrictor, not a vasodilator.

I'm Already Taking Whole Food Supplements!

Clients frequently ask me, if they are already taking whole-food supplements, why would they need herbs?

I've used whole-food supplements and a handful of herbs in clinical practice for more than eight years with great success. So I didn't jump on the bandwagon immediately when I was presented with the idea of using more herbs.

But I've found that using the right types of herbs has been a welcome addition to the Standard Process whole-food nutritional supplements that have been so effective for my clients. (See Part Two on buying and taking herbs.) Through study and practice, I've found that herbs play a unique part in our healing.

Great Economic Reasons to Take Herbs

Let's look at a few reasons why you'll save money and get healthier by using herbs.

1. Herbs help you take control of your own health care. Herbal medicine has always been a strong and viable alternative to pharmaceutical medications. In so many cases, herbal supplements are just as effective, if not more effective than medications.

Additionally, when people begin to look at the idea of taking herbs, they also begin to understand why it's so important to be aware of the types and quality of foods they eat, and the importance of cleaning up their diet and lifestyle by drinking lots of pure water, getting adequate exercise, and eating lots of good quality fruits and vegetables. By adapting a healthier lifestyle, people dramatically reduce the risk of disease.

2. Herbs are simply more cost effective than drugs. And the more you take herbs, the more likely you won't even need drugs.

I see dozens of clients daily, many who have just returned from the drug store. I'm still shocked that some drugs can cost up to $200 a month! Who wouldn't want to seek at least a cheaper (and much safer!) alternative? Health care costs are becoming overwhelming for the average person.

According to author Phyllis Balch, a year's supply of the latest diabetes medication can cost $5,000![37]

While herbs are a better bet, when people purchase herbs, most people shop for the lowest prices. Here's where quality really matters. You do get what you pay for. For example, there is a huge difference between a three dollar bottle of Echinacea and a fifteen dollar bottle! My best advice is to take herbs from a reputable company. See Chapter Six for more information.

Why Take Herbs?

Clients are always asking me about herbs for certain conditions they might have. Here are a few of the funnier examples for which I could not find an herbal solution!:

Girls ask: Is there an herb that will make me tall, blond and thinner?

Guys might ask: Is there an herb that will help me grow hair on my head?

Kids might ask: Is there an herb to make my little brother nicer?

And anyone might ask: Is there an herb that will make me smarter, better looking and rich?

There Are Many Benefits of Herbs

Herbs have literally thousands of uses and are extremely beneficial. Here's a short list of major benefits.

*Tasty herbs are ideal for cooking

*Herbs are fairly easy to obtain

*Herbs are used to prevent disease and maintain health

*Herbs contain nutrients and antioxidants

*Herbs have a long history of safe use

*Herbs are rich in compounds that have wonderful effect on organs and tissues

*Herbs have few if any side effects

Special Needs for Herbs Today

Why the resurgence of herbal therapy? Our country has eaten refined, processed foods and been exposed to toxins that our grandparents never knew. Now we are experiencing diseases that used to be rare such as tuberculosis (TB) and autoimmune diseases. Because of the overuse of antibiotics, that are becoming more and more ineffective, people are searching for better ways to heal their bodies.

It's hard to understand why herbs are so wonderful, effective and absolutely perfect for our bodies unless you understand how our bodies work. Herbs are wonderful and help the body heal in a way that drugs can't. In Chapter One, I mentioned the four stages of disease:

1. Poor digestion
2. A sluggish liver
3. Poor elimination
4. A weakened immune system

45

Let's look at how herbs help to prevent disease.

1. Herbs are great for improving digestion. In fact, traditional herbalists often begin their check up and supplementation with digestion. When digestion is weak, food particles can end up in the blood which causes symptoms of allergies, arthritis, and a weakened immune system. Bitter tonics are bitter tasting herbs (yummm!) that stimulate production of your body's own digestive enzymes. Taken before meals, they increase your body's digestion.

2. Herbs are wonderful for the liver. In Chinese Medicine, there is a saying that "you are only as healthy as your liver." Science has validated this. When a person's liver is healthy, they are much stronger and less likely to get degenerative diseases such as arthritis and cancer. There are many herbs available that support the liver. For example, Milk Thistle, also known as Silymarin, can help to restore and regenerate liver cells.

3. Herbs are great for supporting proper elimination. Traditionally, herbs are superior for toning the entire digestive tract. Here are some herbs used in Standard Process product, **SP Cleanse®:**

Juniper berry powder: diuretic and urinary antiseptic

Red clover flower: cleanses blood and supports immune system

Collinsonia root: increases strength of peristalsis

Burdock root powder: cleanses lymph, and is an antimicrobial

Barley grass powder: source of chlorophyll, a liver cleansing agent

Together these nutrients help support bile production, pull fat from the liver, and break down fat and toxins. Additionally, Cascara helps clear out the bowel and Globe Artichoke stimulates bile and urine flow to cleanse the body.

4. Herbs are great for enhancing a weakened immune system. If you are the one who gets a cold or two every year, you might consider taking herbs. I've had literally hundreds of clients who came in with seriously weakened immune systems. In our office, I've successfully recommended various herbs such as Echinacea which helped tremendously. I learned the hard way to to support my staff and myself with the MediHerb Echinacea Premium. You see, sometimes people came in with conditions such as Strep throat, and they either didn't know at the time or forget to tell us, so we all got Strep throat, too! We don't get caught off guard any more.

Plants not only offer vitamins minerals and trace elements but they also provide nutrients that protect the plant itself from environmental pollution. Lorna Vanderhaeghe in *The Immune System Cure* reports that of necessity, plants are being rediscovered and reconsidered since bacteria are becoming so resistant to antibiotic therapy.[38]

An Herbal Wonder

An ancient effective, yet gentle detoxifier that cleanses body systems and organs, called Essiac, was originally designed for cancer over sixty years ago and is well known as a cancer preventative. Even yeast sensitive people can use this formula. The four herbs contained in this formula are: Sheep Sorrel, Burdock Root, Slippery Elm Bark, and Turkish Rhubarb which have been around for years.

A natural diuretic, this formula boosts the immune system, helps with constipation, purifies the blood and lymph, aids digestion and soothes the entire intestinal tract. For athletes, increases in endurance and strength are reported with decreased recuperation time. It's also an excellent skin moisturizer. Here is a short list of conditions which are helped: arthritis, asthma, allergies, cancer, Chronic Fatigue Syndrome, diabetes, irregularity, Parkinson's disease, swollen ankles, thyroid disorders, ulcers, urinary disorders, varicose veins and warts. (Wow—who wouldn't want to take it?)

Kerry Bone, an expert herbalist, developed a similar herbal formula called Burdock Complex®. Burdock Complex enhances the immune response; supports the body's organs of elimination; supports healthy mucus membranes in the digestive systems; maintains healthy blood, and keeps skin healthy.

Here are the herbs that are contained in the MediHerb Burdock Complex®. (Sometimes the herb Cat's Claw is also included in the original Essiac formulas.)

Burdock Root is best known for its beneficial effect to the skin.

Sheep Sorrel is known for healing a wide variety of skin disorders. It's been shown to strengthen the immune system and is rich in chlorophyll.

Turkish Rhubarb Root has been used in China more than 2,000 years. It has impressive detoxifying properties and is excellent liver cleanser with antibiotic and anti-microbial properties.

Slippery Elm Root has been reported to reduce pain from ulcers because the mucilage coats any area it passes through. Also an antibiotic and anti-microbial, it helps remove toxins from the body.

Other herbs which are recommended for weakened immune system are MediHerb product Astragalus, and Andrographis.

My assistant, Carolyn really loved the MediHerb product combination Albizia and Euphrasia for her symptoms of allergies—it worked great.

Other Great Benefits of Herbs

I've recommended herbs to my clients for several years. Here are some other benefits of herbs and some of the herbs we have used with good results.

5. Herbs also help with energy. Obviously, people use caffeine as an energy booster. But caffeine isn't recommended and it often only masks the real reasons for lack of energy, such as weakened adrenal glands or thyroid, or even anemia. (For more information on how to get more energy, see my book entitled, *Why Am I So Grumpy, Dopey and Sleepy?*) Common herbs that support the adrenal glands, thus giving more energy are the energy promoting ginseng herbs, such as Eleuthero (Siberian Ginseng). Herbs such as Eleuthero help to balance the endocrine system. My clients really like a MediHerb product called Withania for chronic fatigue and stress management.

MediHerb has a product called Thyroid Complex® which we just love. It's not only helped people with energy, but has helped my clients with weight loss as well.

6. Herbs prevent or reduce the risk of heart disease, cancer and diabetes. Garlic, for example, has components that support the body in such a way to prevent all three. Herbs that strengthen the heart are Ginkgo and Hawthorn, and immune system building herbs such as Astragalus and Echinacea help the body avoid serious disease.

Several herbs have an amazing action on the liver. For example, Milk Thistle will actually assist in repairing damaged liver cells. Drugs only tear them down. Other herbs, such as, Globe Artichoke and Dandelion Root, promote bile production.

7. Herbs can help improve your memory. Memory herbs include one of my favorite, a Standard Process product called Ginkgo Synergy®. It increases circulation and thus oxygen to the brain. MediHerb has a product called Bacopa which contains a nice combination of Schisandra, Eleuthero, Bacopa and Rosemary. This combination has helped many of my clients who struggle with Attention Deficit Disorder.

Standard Process has Cayenne Pepper which supports a healthy immune system, being one of the best sources of vitamins C and E. It also supports digestion, circulation and enhances metabolic efficiency.

8. Herbs support the nervous system and can really help with depression. When my mother passed away a few years ago, I really was pleased with the St. John's Wort by Standard Process. It really kept me from depression and since then, hundreds of my clients have given me good reports from taking it. My office manager, Anne really likes a MediHerb product called Nevaton. She reports that it keeps her calm and she sleeps better with it. I also recommend a MediHerb product, Valerian for sleep related problems.

9. Herbs support both male and female endocrine balance. For females, I've used herbs such as Chaste Tree to enhance fertility, support milk production and help relieve symptoms of PMS and menopause. For males, Saw Palmetto has been an incredible source of nutrients for the prostate. Tribulus is the name of a MediHerb product that supports both male and female physiology. MediHerb also carries a Black Cohosh which has helped my clients with such problems as hot flashes, night sweats and vaginal dryness.

Standard Process Palmettoplex® is a great support for the prostate and contains Saw Palmetto Berry Extract, Stinging Nettle Root and Pygeum.

Cramplex is a MediHerb that really helps with menstrual cramping. My assistant, Carolyn uses both Cramplex and Saligesic with great success for her lower back pain. Anne likes the herb Chaste Tree and reports that it helps greatly with her PMS. A client named Karen reported that the MediHerb product Feverfew eliminated the migraine headaches she usually got with her monthly cycle.

10. Herbs support blood sugar levels. We love the MediHerb, Gymnema. It's helped my clients with sugar and carbohydrate cravings, and has also helped to lower surging insulin levels. You'll want to work with your health professional if you are on insulin and begin to take Gymnema.

Here are some general examples of herbs used for various parts of the body:

· **The Digestive System:** Aloe vera, Garlic, Ginger and Peppermint aid digestion. Dandelion and Burdock Root help the gallbladder; Milk Thistle, Globe Artichoke, and Dandelion help the liver; and Aloe, Fennel, Pau d'arco, Slippery Elm and Psyllium help the intestines. The Standard Process product, Gastro-Fiber®, is a great source of Psyllium.

· **The Musculoskeletal System and Hair, Skin and Joints:** Horsetail, Aloe Vera, Alfalfa, Boswellia, Celery and Garlic all support these tissues.

· **The Immune System:** Echinacea, Astragalus, Andrographis, Cat's Claw and Garlic all support the immune system.

· **The Central Nervous System:** Ashwaganda, Siberian Ginseng, Valerian and St. John's Wort have a positive effect on the central nervous system.

· **The Endocrine System:** Ashwaganda, Astragalus, Rehmannia and Licorice all support the adrenal glands. Bladderwrack supports the thyroid gland.

· **The Cardiovascular System:** Garlic, Ginkgo, Cayenne and Hawthorn help the heart and circulation; Cayenne, Hawthorn and Horse Chestnut all help the blood vessels.

How Much Do You Really Know About Herbs?

Some herbs have such unusual names that you wonder how they got them! Take this little quiz that my nephew, David, wrote to see how many you recognize.

You really don't know much about herbs if...

*You think Bacopa sounds like an Island in the Caribbean.

*You think Gota Kola is a Chinese brand of soda.

*You think Tribulus is the name of a great Roman emperor.

*You think Astragalus is the name of a new hair cream for men.

*You think Albizia and Euphrasia are small countries in Eastern Europe.

*You think Cilantro is a large city in Mexico.

*You think Cayenne is the capital of Wyoming.

*You think Chinese Skullcap is head gear for small people.

*You think Pau d'arco was Joan of Arc's third cousin.

*You think Pumaco is an oil company in South America.

*You think Milk Thistle is the milk from a prickly cow!

*You think Ganoderma and Shitake are the names of two famous Indian Chiefs.

*You think Shepherd's Purse is the name of a fashion accessory store.

In spite of their unusual names, though, herbs are quite amazing.

Let's go to Chapter Four to see how herbs compare to drugs.

How Do Herbs Compare to Drugs?

On one hand, we've got a plastic orange bottle with a white top, and a long list of side effects which include dry mouth, seizures and insomnia...your skin may clear up, but did you really need to sleep this week anyway? On the other hand, you've got a plant with generally no side effects. While people may still be debating which came first, the chicken or the egg, in the case of herbs and drugs, herbs came first and because of their safety, they have lasted for centuries.

Did you know that today many of the drugs that we take have ingredients which were extracted from a plant source? The word "drug" comes from the old Dutch word, "drogge" which means "to dry" since pharmacists, physicians and ancient healers often dried plants for use as medicines.[39] However, while the language has stayed the same, the plants have been changed to drugs. There is still a big difference between medicinal drugs and plant herbs.

The word "herb" comes from the Latin word for grass. Herbs have been used for centuries and are still being used today. The World Health Organization reports that of the 119 plant derived pharmaceutical medicines, about 74 percent of these herbs are used today in modern medicine in ways that relate directly with their traditional uses as plant medicines by native cultures.[40]

Most people don't know that prior to the discovery of antibiotics, the now popular herb, Echinacea, was one of the most popular herbal medicines in the U.S. In Chapter Two I showed you the history of herbal medicines, and how long-standing herbal traditions fell by the wayside.

So what's the difference? Are drugs the "wonder" agents of the modern centuries? Are they good for us or not?

To fully understand the difference between pharmaceutical drugs and plant herbs, it helps to step back and look at the difference between synthetic and natural vitamins.

The Whole-Food Difference

There has always been a debate about the types of supplements available. As I wrote in my book, *Why Do I Need Whole-Food Supplements,* there are three types of supplement processing methods: natural, synthetic, and crystalline. Natural, whole-supplements are whole foods with just the water and fiber removed. These are the most natural form of supplementing your diet, and you can generally tell a natural supplement because it will list the food sources from which these supplements were obtained. Examples are: wheat germ, brewer's yeast, acerola cherries, etc.

Synthetic vitamins are toxic to the body and can actually **cause** vitamin deficiencies. Just compare an orange to ascorbic acid or vitamin C. The orange has the full vitamin C complex with all of the enzymes, coenzymes, antioxidants, trace elements, activators, and other unknown factors that cause the vitamin to work. Ascorbic acid, which is commonly sold as vitamin C, is only one part of this once whole food!

According to Dr. Royal Lee, **vitamins that are isolated or synthesized in the laboratory are not natural, act as a drug, are toxic, and cause imbalance in the body chemistry.** Natural vitamins are foods and they only work as nutrition when still contained in the whole complex, with all of the other synergists found in nature.[41]

In other words, you can't take a complex apart and expect it to work the way God designed it. Once it has been separated, the components are missing. If your body already has the cofactors to recombine and process ascorbic acid, you could experience some improvement for a time. If you don't, the ascorbic acid won't benefit you. The symptoms you were trying to eliminate will return, and you will end up with a vitamin C deficiency.

Synthetic vitamins are usually much cheaper than natural supplements since natural supplements involve growing whole food substances. Synthetic supplements can come from many sources, including by products of various petro chemical companies. So taking one or more isolated vitamins can actually create an imbalance of vitamins which is worse than a deficiency.

How Are Most Drugs Made?

To understand the difference between herbs and drugs, **think of drugs as working in a similar manner as synthetic vitamins and herbs working in a similar manner as the whole-food supplements.**

Look at how drugs are made. Rather than using a whole plant, drug manufacturers isolate, and extract components. Entire drug industries are based on the ability to isolate chemicals originally in herbs and make them into drugs. But when parts are isolated, there can be problems, since herbs are designed to work as a whole.

According to Master Herbalist Louise Tenney, isolating what we consider the most active compound of a plant doesn't mean that it's the healing agent. Louise Tenney wrote:

> When you eliminate certain plant ingredients in order to isolate what is considered the active principle of an herb, you can destroy the synergistic or balancing effect of the whole medicinal plant.[42]

Our bodies know how to take the nutrition from herbs and disregard the rest, without any side effects. Unfortunately, this is not the same with drugs, which are foreign to our bodies. This explains why drugs, while somewhat effective in eliminating symptoms, usually cause many side effects.

A Long-Standing Debate

The argument between drug companies and natural healers has gone on throughout our history. Herbalists believe that nature provides ingredients in herbs to counteract powerful ingredients in them. These ingredients act as counterbalances so when you use herbs in their complete form, they are safe and effective.

For example, the herb Lobelia is criticized as toxic because it contains alkaloids which when acting alone are central nervous system depressants that can cause a coma or death.

According to herbalist Mark Pedersen, with the proper dosage, these alkaloids relax the body and make them useful for treating asthma. He explains that the safe dispensing of Lobelia requires professional supervision. But who is qualified to ingest Lobelia safely? Anyone who has ever vomited. He explains that nature built an overdose prevention that causes an excessive amount to be expelled by the overwhelming need to vomit.[43]

Herbs are great communicators; they warn you ahead of time of possible danger!

Another example that Mark gives is the drug Digitalis which comes from a plant called foxglove. An overdose of Digitalis is apparent when the patient experiences heart arrhythmias, which are side effects of the drug. Long before Digitalis was developed, herbalists used Foxglove to treat dropsy for congestive heart failure. However, Mark explains that the herbalist knew of a potential overdose of Foxglove when the patient complained of irritation in the stomach which always happened before the arrythmias. Nature provides protection against an overdose of Foxglove by warning him to stop taking the herb (irritation) or he will get sicker (arrhythmia).[44]

The reason this causes side effects is that herbs contain numerous components including minerals, oils, vitamins and bioflavonoids which support the herb's properties. They also balance the herb so that isolated compounds normally taken in a whole herb are safe, but could be toxic when isolated and synthesized.

So many drugs are derived from plants. Today in the U.S., nearly 25% of all prescriptions contain ingredients derived from plants. Here are a few common examples from Earl Mindell in his book, *Earl Mindell's New Herb Bible*:[45]

Aspirin is a chemical imitation of salicin found in white willow bark.

Reserpine, a blood pressure medicine, is actually an ancient remedy from India derived from an Asian shrub.

Quinine, a famous malaria treatment, and quinidine, an antiarrhythmic medication, are made from the bark of the cinchona tree.

A Comparison of Herbs and Drugs

In the last chapter, I gave several benefits of herbs and said that herbs helped people have control of their health and are more cost effective. Let's review and contrast the benefits of herbs that I listed earlier with drugs (see page 44).

Tasty herbs are ideal for cooking. When was the last time you used Tylenol in your lasagne recipe?

Herbs are easy to obtain. Drugs can be purchased over-the-counter, (or on the street, but I wouldn't know where!) but obtaining prescription drugs can be difficult.

Herbs are used to prevent disease and maintain health. Drugs do not act in the same way as herbs do. Drugs "prevent" disease by covering up or suppressing symptoms. Drug therapies are not very effective to treat diseases caused by poor diet, stress and toxins. Plant compounds are shown to help the immune system fight cancer, and destroy viruses.

Let's review great reasons to take herbs that I presented in the previous chapter which are far better served with herbal therapy as opposed to drug therapy (see page 45).

1. Herbs are great for improving digestion.
2. Herbs are wonderful for the liver.
3. Herbs are great for supporting proper elimination.
4. Herbs are great for enhancing a weakened immune system.

5. Herbs also help with energy.

6. Herbs reduce the risk of heart disease, cancer and diabetes.

7. Herbs can help improve your memory.

8. Herbs support both male and female endocrine balance.

Herbs contain nutrients and antioxidants. Drugs do not contain nutrients or antioxidants.

Herbs have a long history of safe use. Drugs do not have a history of safe use, and in fact, have been known to have side effects. (See Chapter Five.)

Herbs are rich in compounds that have wonderful effect on organs and tissues. Drugs are known toxins.

Herbs have few if any side effects. I discuss the safety issue of herbs in Chapter Seven, but generally speaking herbs are very safe when used properly. Drugs have considerable, known side effects. (See Chapter Five.)

Herbal Therapies Challenged

I've read articles written by medical experts explaining that alternative health care which uses nutritional supplements, for example, is "quackery." Yet, according to our government, orthodox medicine is 80% unproven!

The Government Publication #PB286-929 says,

> It has been estimated that only 10-20 percent of all procedures currently used in medical practice have been shown to be efficacious by controlled trial.

Certainly, there is a place for medical doctors and surgery for life-threatening situations. But did you know that whenever there were strikes by doctors in 1973, 1976 and 1978, according to researcher Louise Tenney, their absence decreased death rates?[46]

Also in 1973, there was a 29-day physicians strike in Great Britain and 50% fewer deaths were reported.[47]

According to the U.S. Food and Drug Association (FDA), medical errors are the eighth leading cause of death among Americans!

Herbs Just Don't Get Any Respect!

According to the authors of *Smart Medicine,* almost all of the current research validating herbal medicine has been done in Germany, Japan, China, Taiwan and Russia. In spite of the fact that this research is solid, scientific and start-of-the-art, the U.S. Food and Drug Administration (FDA) which licenses all new drugs in the U.S. does not recognize or accept findings from across the sea. Government agencies and physicians want American scientific studies before they recognize the effectiveness of plants as medicine. So herbal medicine in the U.S. doesn't have the same respect as it does in other countries.[48]

However, most reputable American herb manufacturers stay current with this scientific research in China, Japan, Europe and Germany.

Additionally, in the U.S., there is no national licensing or certification for herbalists. (However, there are reputable licensing organizations for certified health professionals using herbs, mentioned in Chapter Eleven.)

Herbs, Drugs and the Law

In his book, *Nutritional Herbology,* Mark Pedersen, reports that the legal definition of a drug in the U.S. is anything which affects the structure or function of the body and is sold to cure, prevent or treat a disease. Foods are not drugs unless they are sold for these reasons. Otherwise, they would be considered drugs since they do affect structure and function of the body.[49]

He further explains that in order for a drug manufacturer to make claims that a substance will act on the symptoms of a disease, the substance must be put through rigorous testing which could cost millions. These laws were originally instated because of the problems with chemical drugs which have harmful side effects. While these laws do protect the public against chemicals which don't work or have serious side effects, they also limit the use of natural herbs as medicines.

Here's why. Drug companies rely on patents to recover the millions of dollars they spend to test a drug. So they are only interested in chemicals which can be patented, not foods or herbs such as garlic.

Garlic has been tested for years. In spite of the fact that garlic has antibiotic effects, it can't be marketed for these purposes. In order to sell garlic as an antibiotic a company would have to pass FDA testing requirements to prove it "safe." But how would the company recover its investment? Anyone can purchase garlic at the grocery store. So drug researchers isolate chemicals which can be patented.

Herbs are not as profitable as drugs. Even if an herb is known to be beneficial, it can't be sold as a drug without the FDA approval. It's this extensive and expensive testing by the FDA that causes the cost of prescriptions to skyrocket.

When Should I Use Drugs Versus Herbs?

While herbal formulas are wonderful healing agents, there are still times when it's appropriate to take drugs. If you are experiencing a condition that is an immediate threat to your life, consult your doctor. Here are some symptoms that require immediate medical attention:[50]

*Chest pain, or pain that radiates down the left arm and chest

*Suspected bone fractures

*Suspected poisoning from foods or chemicals

*Suspected stroke or heart palpitations or severe high blood pressure

*High fever or loss of consciousness

*Severe burns or infections

*Uncontrolled bleeding, diarrhea or vomiting

*Severe pain

If a minor ailment doesn't respond to your herbal treatment within two weeks, see your doctor.

Chapter Five

How Do Drugs Work?

Recently, one of my clients went to her doctor about a rash. She read the label on a drug he had prescribed which said that after taking it, she could have kidney failure within a year! And people are concerned about taking natural herbs or whole-food supplements. Go figure!

Yet what do drugs do to your body? Most of my clients are usually unaware of the damaging effect of many medications on their liver.

What About Side Effects?

Phyllis Balch reports that 400,000 people die of predictable side effects of prescribed drugs, taken with the hope that their potential benefit outweighs the known risks. Thousands of others die due to unpredictable side effects of prescribed drugs. It's not surprising, really. A textbook for pharmacists says that if a drug is stated to have no side effects, then it is strongly suspected it has no central benefit.[51]

When pharmaceutical drugs cause symptom relief, at the same time, they can bombard the liver. That's why so many doctors need to "monitor" liver enzymes, to indicate possible liver damage. This is scary since by the time the liver enzymes show up high on a blood test, nearly 70% of the damage is already done!

A recent overview of 39 studies by researchers at the University of Toronto showed that pharmaceutical drugs are between the fourth and sixth leading cause of deaths in the United States, even when taken as properly prescribed by a doctor.[52] **Of course, people usually forget that herbs have been around since the beginning of civilization, and drugs**

as we are using them have been around for about sixty or seventy years!

People accept drugs prescribed by a doctor without any thought and assume they are safe. But every drug has serious side effects and thousands of people are affected by drugs. In another article in the *Washington Post* entitled, "Correctly Prescribed Drugs Take Heavy Toll," Rick Weiss wrote:[53]

> More than 2 million Americans become seriously ill every year because of toxic reactions to correctly prescribed medicines taken properly, and 106,000 die from those reactions, a new study concludes. That surprisingly high number makes drug side effects at least the sixth...most common cause of death in this country.

Drug companies spend billions of dollars on television advertisements, and they downplay the side effects. It would be better if commercials dramatized the side effects as well as the benefits. For example, you see a handsome man taking medicine for his allergies. Then you see him running to the nearest bathroom when the diarrhea hits!

Drugs are toxic to our bodies and they accumulate in organs and tissues since they are so hard to eliminate. This can lead to other diseases. Drugs work faster and are more potent than herbs. However, in their transition, the body now identifies them as foreign substances. That's why drugs cause side effects.

Dr. John Lee reports that pain drugs such as Nonsteroidal anti-inflammatory drugs (NSAIDS) cause considerable sickness due to their side effects of indigestion, intestinal bleeding, kidney dysfunction, hypertension problems, and precipitation of heart failure.[54]

According to Dr. Marcus Laux, Aspirin and the family of NSAIDs are estimated to be responsible for 20,000 deaths each year and 125,000 hospitalizations, largely as a result of gastrointestinal ulceration and bleeding.[55]

In contrast, herbs not only alleviate the symptoms, but target the root cause and promote healing.

Check the Side Effects of Your Medications

After a new client visits me, occasionally they might call me and report that since taking the supplements I recommended, they now have some type of symptom. After playing detective, in nearly every case, we have discovered that it was never my supplements, but there were other issues. For example, sometimes they were taking medicinal drugs which have numerous side effects. Often, they have compromised digestion and they lack the proper enzymes to digest anything. And occasionally, they were simply catching a cold or flu and didn't realize it until they had full-blown symptoms.

The first thing I would recommend that you do, if you experience any type of unusual symptom such as dizziness, headache, nausea, and so on is to check all of your pharmaceutical drugs for the list of their side effects. (You may need reading glasses and/or a magnifying glass!) I highly recommend that you read about the side effects of any drugs you are currently taking in a PDR (Physician's Desk Reference), and see what it is doing to you in other parts of your body. For example, the headache medicine may be causing diarrhea, or the pill you take for your acid indigestion may be causing aches and pain in your joints!

Look up every drug that you take—even, "safe, over-the-counter" drugs. (After reading this chapter, you might wonder if there is such a thing!)

Recently I was reminded about this when I read an article by Dr. Bruce West in his newsletter about a woman who came to him with a diagnosis of Parkinson's. She was taking drugs for Parkinson's that were not effective, and were causing even more strong side effects. His investigation revealed that a drug that she had been taking for 10 years for high blood pressure was the cause of her Parkinson's. After six months off of this drug, her Parkinson's disappeared![56]

So many people end up on what Dr. Earl Mindell calls the "drug windmill." For example, a fairly healthy fifty-something male named Bob sees his doctor and, except for some heartburn, gets a clean bill of health. However, he also gets a prescription for heartburn such as Tagamet. Bob now has joint pain, so he take something for pain, such as Tylenol. Unfortunately, Bob likes to have a drink after work to unwind and he is not aware that mixing Tylenol and alcohol can cause severe liver damage. He also is unaware that the joint pain came from taking Tagamet! Later, Bob keeps getting colds and sinus problems from a toxic liver, so the doctor prescribes antibiotics and allergy drugs. Now he feels really miserable![57] But what can he do?

If he had a "nutrition-minded" healthcare professional, he could get some help with his digestion so he wouldn't need the Tagamet. I would suggest digestive enzymes such as Standard Process Zypan, Multizyme or MediHerb Digest, as appropriate. When his digestion improves, he may not have joint pain, so he wouldn't need the Tylenol. In the meantime, however, herbal (MediHerb Milk Thistle) or nutritional support (Standard Process Livaplex) would help his liver. Echinacea would support his immune system without side effects. With the right dietary changes and supplementation, Bob could finally get better instead of worse!

Drugs Can Cause Vitamin Deficiencies

Cholesterol medications are called statin drugs. While they do lower cholesterol, unfortunately, they hurt the liver and deplete a nutrient that your heart depends on for great health which is called Co-Q10. Without CoQ10, your heart would stop beating. The drug manufacturers know that statin drugs cause this deficiency, yet there is never any mention of taking this supplement along with the drug (instead of it!)

Many drugs interact with nutrients in the body, often causing further depletion. For example, according to Bruce West:

*Taking estrogen depletes your body of vitamin F, vitamins B1, 2, 3, 6 and 12; vitamin C; minerals and amino acids.

*Taking antibiotics deplete the B complex vitamins and vitamin K.

*Taking blood pressure and cholesterol drugs deplete coenzyme-Q10 and melatonin.

*Taking diabetes drugs deplete CoQ10, B vitamins, B12, and vitamin F.[58]

Drugs for hyperactivity are rampant in this country. According to Bruce West, one in 30 children, from ages five to nineteen take Ritalin. These drugs set children up for a lifetime of emotional problems and can turn them into drug addicts.[59]

Most of these conditions could be helped through diet, exercise and natural supplements, including vitamins and herbs with no side effects.

Why Are Some Drugs Still on the Market?

You might wonder why Acetaminophen, which is responsible for thousands of deaths, is still on the market, but the herb Ephedra, which is responsible for ten deaths, has been taken off the market.

Unfortunately, there is no central governmental control for evaluating the benefits of herbs. Additionally, there is a bias against herbal medicine by the medical association which makes the government less tolerant towards herbs. The FDA allows some risks associated with prescription drugs because they also have proven benefits (again, in spite of the side effects.) However, since herbs may be seen to have little benefit (which is not true), any risk, whatever size, seems unacceptable.

Americans spend trillions of dollars on health care, yet we are still dying from heart disease, cancer and diabetes. If prescription drugs worked, shouldn't we have the best health statistics?

The Philosophy of Drug Therapy

As I mentioned earlier, there are times when drugs are required to save lives. But think about how drugs are recommended so commonly for things that are related to nutritional or lifestyle factors.

A common example is taking a drug for leg cramps which is often a deficiency in either calcium, magnesium, Vitamin B complex or Vitamin E complex. Drugs and surgery have their place in healing in the short term; but when we use these drugs to heal something that was supposed to be healed with natural agents, it can open the door to more problems.

Have you noticed that most of the time when you are prescribed a drug, you have to take it for your lifetime? Don't you wonder about that? I mean, if it really "fixed" you, why can't you get off it at some time? Aren't you somewhat uncomfortable when told you need to stay on a drug "for the rest of your life"?

Drugs don't cure anything. They are designed to give you symptomatic relief only. This isn't always bad, since drugs can, for example, help to lower cholesterol. But most people don't understand that by suppressing some type of action, in this case, stopping the liver from making cholesterol, they are affecting something else. In this case, it affects your body's ability to use fats. This causes an essential fatty acid deficiency, which can further cause such serious problems as memory loss, immune dysfunction, and hormone imbalance. So drugs never fix or cure anything without affecting something else—which is why there are so many side effects.

Think about it. Why would the drug companies want you to be permanently "fixed?" The drug industry is a billion dollar industry. They would be out a lot of money if you really became well and stopped requiring their drugs. But our bodies pay a price when we take these drugs long term.

Are Drugs Really Scientifically-Proven"?

Dr. Bruce West quoted a recent issue of a *British Medical Journal* which said that drug companies can pretty much get the results they want. His conclusion was that lots of "scientifically proven" medicine is hogwash. Studies are used to make sales. Even if a drug shows to be dangerous, every attempt is made to disprove it. Fully 70% of all trials in esteemed medical journals (the gold standard) are funded by the company producing the drug![60]

Here's an example of a heart medication which had unusual side effects—Viagra. When drug manufacturers saw the side effects. they were quick to market this new drug. The latest reports show that taking Viagra with certain heart medications can be fatal. And no one knows about the long-term safety and effectiveness of this drug, while circulatory herbs such as Ginkgo, Garlic, Cayenne and Hawthorne can be beneficial with no side effects.

In his newsletter, Dr. Marcus Laux quoted a senior executive of GlaxoSmithKline, one of the largest drug companies in the world, saying that prescription medicines do not work for most people and that fewer than half of the patients prescribed some of the most expensive drugs actually derived any benefit from them. This is an open secret within the drug companies, but the admission by such a high-level executive made big news. He added that statistically, more than 90 percent of drugs work in only 30-50 percent of people. His conclusion is that drug-based symptom relief does not work with the body's intelligence and more often works against it.[61]

The FDA and the Herb Stevia

How foods are approved is quite an interesting story. I think Donna Gates gives another good example about Stevia in her book, *The Stevia Story.*

While Americans wait for a "safe" sweetener, people in South America have enjoyed a safe, natural sweetener that is calorie-free for years. This sweetener is a South American herb called Stevia and is estimated to be several hundred times sweeter than sugar, so a little goes a long way.

The good news is that it has no dangerous side effects. Numerous studies proving its safety have been done in Japan. In the 1960s, the Japanese either banned or strictly regulated all artificial sweeteners. They soon discovered Stevia and considered it an ideal replacement for both sugar and its synthetic substitutes. Stevia products quickly caught on. By 1988, they represented approximately 41% of the market share of sweet substances consumed in Japan. In addition to widespread use as a tabletop sweetener, Stevia is used by the Japanese to sweeten a variety of food products, including ice cream, bread, candies, pickles, seafood, vegetables, and soft drinks.

Since I tell my clients about Stevia, they always ask me why they can't find it on grocery store shelves. Even though Stevia can now be legally marketed as a dietary supplement, any mention of its possible use as a sweetener or in tea is still strictly prohibited.

Even though Stevia has been proven safe in many countries, since the mid-1980s, the U.S. Food and Drug Administration labeled Stevia an "unsafe food additive" and went to extensive lengths to keep it off the U.S. market.

Judging from the extensive measures the FDA has used to keep Americans in the dark about Stevia, you might think it was a dangerous drug. Although it has been used by millions of people around the world, in some places for hundreds of years, there have been no negative side effects.

By denying Stevia the official GRAS or "Generally Regarded As Safe" status, the FDA was able to put Stevia in the "food additive" category, which requires that it undergo substantial scientific study prior to marketing.[62]

This makes you wonder how drugs make it to market in the first place if they have to be approved as safe. Notice the warning on the back of the Saccharin packet: "Use of this product may be hazardous to your health. This product contains saccharin, which has been determined to cause cancer in laboratory animals." This product hasn't been determined safe, yet it's in everything!

Donna Gates explains that since Stevia is a sweetener, it's considered an additive with a particularly high potential for mass consumption, so it necessitates "special scrutiny." Never mind that this requirement was totally relaxed when the FDA approved aspartame, (an artificial sweetener found in most diet drinks) which has not been proven safe.[63] However, manufacturers in the U.S. are still restricted from using Stevia as an additive.

Why Don't We Know About Herbs?

I have file drawers of health testimonies of my clients, but you'll probably never hear about them on the nightly news. Don't you wonder why we rarely hear about exceptional cases of natural healing?

Unfortunately, we don't get the full truth on the television news, because drug companies spend billions of dollars to fund television programs. Did you ever notice that just after the "health" news there are several drug advertisements? The media wouldn't report on the incredible benefits of St. John's Wort for depression, for example, when during that news cast, there was a drug advertisement for Prozac.

I encourage you to consider going to a natural healthcare professional if you are taking many medications. Perhaps with the right diet, exercise, nutritional supplements and herbs, you may work with your doctor to wean off some of the medications you are taking that may be hurting you more than you know.

Let's now go to Part Two to learn more about how to buy herbs.

PART TWO

How to Buy and Take Herbs

Chapter Six

Are All Herbal Supplements Alike?

You may be like so many of my clients who have a cabinet full of a variety of herbal supplements and vitamins, but you still don't feel any better. Perhaps the fact that you are taking the herbs that your Aunt Mabel grew and sold out of her basement might have something to do with it!

How much difference in quality is there between different brands? Quality is determined by many factors: growing, harvesting, and processing—but it's hard to know the difference when staring at the labels of the hundreds of bottles on the health food store shelf.

Types of Herbal Supplements

There are all kinds of supplements around and I've discovered that not all herbal products are the same. Not all herbs contain the same levels of active constituents. Not all herbs are grown or harvested or dried or stored in the same way. And the standards of growers, suppliers, and manufacturers are not the same. You may not be getting what you think you are getting!

In this chapter, we'll look at the different ways that herbs can vary, which will help explain why some herbs work and why some don't seem to do anything.

In today's unregulated supplement market, it might not surprise you that independent tests have found over and over that most herbs don't contain what their labels say they contain. A testing laboratory in White Plains, NY, tested 11 brands of Echinacea and found many inconsistencies. Twenty-five percent had some type of problem, ranging from containing less than the label said, the wrong ingredient, or an inability to properly break down as promised.[64]

Drug companies by law must prove that their drugs work (even if there are accompanying side effects and their "studies" are questionable.) However, since herbal supplements are not regulated by the FDA, herbal supplement manufacturers don't have to do this because they can't claim that herbs cure anything. Anyone can sell herbs.

We may see more legislation in the future. In the meantime, telling the difference between a good supplement and an inferior one is often difficult.

So what makes a good herbal product?

High Standards Make Quality Products

A great example of a good herbal product is the Australian company, MediHerb, which I use in my office and is sold only to licensed, certified health professionals. Herbal expert Kerry Bone is the MediHerb Founder and Director of Research and Development. Kerry explains their standard of Good Manufacturing Practice (GMP) is legally required for the manufacture of herbal products in many countries including Australia, Japan, Canada and Germany. Pharmaceutical GMP is a fail-safe standard of quality control which defines a number of procedures including:

The validation of equipment

The documented standard operating procedures

The control of the manufacturing environment, air and water

The quarantining and identification and testing of raw material

The testing for shelf life

Herbal manufacturing under GMP is essential because the issues are more complex than those for conventional drugs. According to Bone, there are several reasons why this is so.[65]

1. Herbs are biologically defined, living entities, unlike drugs. So they could be incorrectly identified, such as the wrong name or wrong species.

2. Herbs may vary in phytochemical content, which could have an impact on their safety and effectiveness.

3. Just as people come with a history, so do herbs. Herbs may be contaminated with toxic minerals, or grown in a field with pesticides which all have an impact on content and quality.

4. How were they harvested, dried and stored? Different manufacturers may not be as careful in each of these processes as others are.

5. Once the herbs are in the factory, how are they extracted and processed into tablets? The processing may enhance or impair their safety and effectiveness.

6. Finally, how stable are they? The stability of an herb greatly impacts its shelf life.

A great deal of expertise and hard work is needed in order to meet these high GMP standards.

Cold Percolation is the Best

According to Bone, the 1:2 Cold Percolation method is unlike any other herbal extraction processes. In this process, no heat or concentration is used, both of which may cause damage to the delicate plant material. The greatest care is taken to prevent any contamination from outside sources throughout the extraction process. Here are some interesting facts about their manufacturing conditions:

*All of their extraction equipment is built from stainless steel.

*Air used in the manufacturing process is thoroughly cleansed using pharmaceutical standard filtering units.

*All process water used in extraction is purified by reverse osmosis.

To date, MediHerb has quantified the actions of over 70 herbs through their "quantified activity" program. To their knowledge such a program has never been undertaken in Australia, nor has it been matched anywhere in the world. Each batch of tablets is tested for disintegration, weight uniformity, and active constituents.

What's Really in Your Herbal Supplement?

To get the best results, you have to use the best herbs available. Organically-grown herbs contain considerably more nutrition and phytochemicals than the typical herbs that are sold over the counter. Few companies are willing to do the extra work required in organic growing.

Additionally, some companies quote the studies to support the use of their herbs in their marketing material, but when they make the product, they don't use the same extracts in their products. Some companies use the extracts in their products, but not at the right doses.

Many clients have come to my office carrying a bag of herbs that they have been taking, boasting that their Echinacea only cost them $3.99 through their latest vitamin mail order catalog. Unfortunately, they also come in with compromised immune systems, and everything else that comes with it such as sore joints and fatigue. My question is, if their Echinacea is so good, why aren't they in better health?

For example, I use the MediHerb product Echinacea Premium. It's so effective, that it takes about 15 of a health food store's "garden variety" to be as therapeutic as one of the Echinacea Premium, which contains Echinacea angustifolia roots which are more potent than the leaves.

There are many problems with the way herbal supplements are often produced in this country.

1. Most herbal tablets are made from powdered, dried herbs or poor quality dried extracts which means they are less potent.

2. Not all herbal manufacturers ensure that the finished tablet is as good as the liquid extracts and that the entire

phytochemical profile of the starting herb has been maintained.

3. Not all herbal manufacturers use the optimal method of low temperatures under vacuum. This step minimizes the exposure of chemicals in the herbal mix to the damaging effects of heat and oxidation.

4. Herbal products can be contaminated with heavy metals or microbial contaminants. Since plants come from nature, herbal raw materials carry a microbial burden which needs to be addressed during processing. Not all manufacturers deal properly with these bacteria. A common practice of manufacturers is to sterilize their herbs which produces an inferior product.

5. Herbal products may be contaminated with conventional drugs. Or, there could be contamination of a safe herb with a toxic herb, for example, digitalis (foxglove leaves) found among symphytum (comfrey leaves).[66]

Following the GMP in a well regulated environment should eliminate the possibility of contamination of drugs and microbes.[67]

6. Many herbal products in the market place just don't work because manufacturers don't hire practicing clinical herbalists. Rather, they make formulas based on what seems to be the most popular herbs at the time, not on what is scientifically proven to be the most effective. Only a handful of the herbal products available were designed by practicing herbalists. Most herbal products are designed by researchers. They are not the herbalists who have actually practiced with herbs, so they don't have any practical experience. This makes customers guinea pigs!

In an attempt to protect consumers from products that don't contain what's on the label and for safety and quality issues, the U. S. FDA is preparing to issue a set of guidelines for dietary supplements called Current Good Manufacturing Practices, or CGMPs. These guidelines will establish requirements regarding the manufacturing, packaging, labeling, testing, quality control and storage of dietary supplements. In the meantime, you need to understand these quality issues. Perhaps the most important, though, is the issue of substitution.

7. Some manufacturers substitute one herb for another. If an herb appears to have "high levels of the active ingredient" on the label, but it has a cheap price, it's probably a substitution and is far less effective. Some examples of substitution are:

a. Substituting the wrong plant part within a species.

Bone gives the example of a woman who was taking Golden Seal but it had no effect on her allergies. When she brought in the bottle, he found that she was using Golden Seal leaf, not the root. The part of the plant that is most beneficial for allergies is the root.

Herbal manufacturers from China, for example, have been known to keep the best parts of Panax Ginseng (the root) for their use and export the cheapest part (the root hairs) to the U.S. or other countries. Root hairs have very little activity and are not the preferred plant part. (That's why the Chinese get better results from taking herbs!)

b. Substituting a less active subspecies or variety of plant. Bone gives an example of Thyme, which has at least five different subspecies. But only one subspecies, Thyme vulgaris thymoliferum, has high levels of the active phenol content. If the manufacturer doesn't test their herbs properly, they would not be aware of this, and they may be using one of the other four subspecies which produces little or no effect.

b. Substituting a related plant of the same genus. Some plants may have different species that are similar in action, such as Willow Bark, so it doesn't matter as much if you substitute a related plant. But, for example, if you substitute Echinacea pallida for Echinacea angustifolia, it is not acceptable and won't give the same effect.

c. Substituting an unrelated plant for another plant.
This means the plant looks like another plant, but they are completely unrelated and act differently. In some cases the substitution is ineffective, but other cases could be more serious. For example, substituting Teucrium species (Germander) for Scutellaria lateriflora (Skullcap). Bone points out that sometimes toxicity is attributed to Skullcap, when in fact it's actually Germander which could be toxic to the liver.[68]

The only way to know what is really in a plant is with a process such as the one MediHerb uses called Thin Layer Chromatography. (See Kerry Bone's book, *The Principles and Practice of Phytotherapy* for further information.)

Standardization

Herbal products are everywhere, but the quality of these products varies greatly. It used to be that you didn't know what you were getting. But today's manufacturing steps are sophisticated and a process called "standardization" is popular. Standardization is a quality control measure designed to ensure batch-to-batch consistency.

Standardization also allows researchers to conduct scientific studies to determine the therapeutic effects of herbs. Identifying the active ingredients and marker compounds helps us know that these herbs have "active" constituents. Herbs quoted in scientific journals are done with standardized extracts. The best studies are those that are tested and proven to have benefits in human trials.

Standardized also means that each dose contains a precise amount of one or more of the herb's active compounds. These are usually described as a percentage of the weight of the herb. Feverfew is standardized for a constituent called parthenolide.

However, one problem with standardization is that it doesn't always guarantee results. Perhaps the label on the herb St. John's Wort indicates "standardized to hypercins." It means that the extract was tested and found to contain a specified amount of those ingredients. However, the hypercins are only the marker, not necessarily the "active" ingredient. So standardization doesn't guarantee that the herb will work especially if the active ingredient is a different component.

Additionally, just because a product is labeled, "standardized," there is no guarantee that the label is correct because standardization is voluntary for manufacturers.

Also, tests of products on the shelf show that some supplements don't contain the levels which they are supposed to contain according to the label.

A recent study in the British journal *The Lancet,* reported that some ginseng formulations contained no active ingredients at all![69]

Some companies misuse the word "standardized" to mean that their capsules weigh the same every time, not that they contain the same amount of active ingredient.

Standardization is only possible when an herb's active ingredients are identified and easily measured. That's why you should buy herbs from established companies like MediHerb who have established reputations. They are more likely to have quality control measures in place.

Labeling Deceptions

There are many misleading labels; what's on the label isn't always what's in the pill! In fact, if people really followed "truth in labeling" some labels might say, "This herb really has nothing significant in it. We just hope it doesn't hurt you!"

Often it's hard to read the label, and labels can be deceptive. Also, the levels of "active" ingredients can vary from batch to batch. So the quality of herbal supplements can vary. Herbs like ginkgo or ginseng have thousands of active compounds and they vary from plant to plant, season to season. Researchers are not always certain which compounds are the "active" ingredients for many herbal products.

Learn to read labels. By reading the fine print you can spot inconsistencies or inaccuracies. The FDA requires that manufacturers of botanical product labels also list both names. If the herbal supplement doesn't list the scientific name as well as the popular name of the herb, don't buy it.

How To Read a Label

A product label is often your only guide to the quality, strength and efficacy of a product. So it's important to know how to interpret the label on an herbal supplement. Here are some things to know:

Normally, with a standardized label, you'll see the name of the compound the standardization is based on, and the percentage of that compound the extract contains. You'll see the ratio, weight, and number of capsules. You will also see the recommended daily doses. The manufacturer should provide their name, address and website as well.

Some herbal products contain a laundry list of herbs that are considered "proprietary" which means that the manufacturer is the only one who knows the formula. They can brag, "This product contains 12 immune-system building herbs." But by this labeling, you have no idea what amount of each herb is in the product.

I'll use the example of a MediHerb label because these are the herbal supplements that I've used in my practice. A MediHerb label provides full disclosure of all ingredients in a consistent, clear and concise manner to pharmaceutical GMP (Good Manufacturing Process) standards.

The Supplement Facts label on page 81 summarizes what you should look for on an herbal tablet label and describes the key elements.

1. Common Name Many herbs have the same or similar common names; therefore it is important to also list the botanical name to avoid confusion.

2. Plant Part Using the correct plant part is crucial since different plant parts can have varying or no effectiveness. For example, Dandelion Root supports liver function and Dandelion Leaf stimulates healthy urine flow.

3. Extract Ratio This indicates the strength of the extract. The number on the left represents the amount of the herb and the number on the right represents the amount of extract. For example, a 4:1 ratio means 4 kilograms of herb are extracted to make 1 kilogram of extract.

4. Extract Different preparation types are sometimes used. It's important to understand the type of preparation being used. MediHerb uses liquid extracts to manufacture their tablets.

5. Botanical Name The botanical name is essential for determining identity and therefore effectiveness. The FDA requires supplement labels to include the scientific name of herbs used, as well as the name of the part of the plant used. If the manufacturer can't list the scientific name of an herb, how can you trust them to produce herbs properly?

6. Quantity of Starting Material. This states the quantity of dried herb equivalent used in each tablet.

7. Quantity of Extract This states the quantity of extract used in the tablet.

8. Identified & Quantified Active Constituent. This represents the quality of an extract as a specific active compound.

9. Table Excipients. An excipient is the "glue" that holds the tablet together. MediHerb uses a range of low allergenic and pharmaceutical grade excipients in the manufacture of its tablet range. These excipients are carefully chosen using experienced gained from 10 years of manufacturing herbal tablets and are necessary to aid in the manufacturing process and to allow ease of swallowing.

For example, hypromellose is used as a film coating on most MediHerb tablets. Here are some advantages of it:

*It makes the tablet more resistant to dust formation in the packaging.

*When the tablet surface is wet in the mouth, a lubricant mucilagenous layer is formed on the tablet which makes swallowing easier.

*An inner layer hides any unpleasant tastes that are found in many herbal products.

*It enhances the stability of a product by forming a barrier to the external environment.

10. An expiration date. For example, on a MediHerb product box you'll see an expiration date.

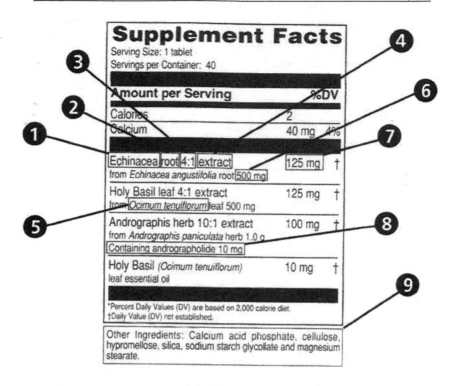

Supplement Facts

Serving Size: 1 tablet
Servings per Container: 40

Amount per Serving		%DV
Calories	2	
Calcium	40 mg	4%
Echinacea root 4:1 extract from *Echinacea angustifolia* root 500 mg	125 mg	†
Holy Basil leaf 4:1 extract from *Ocimum tenuiflorum* leaf 500 mg	125 mg	†
Andrographis herb 10:1 extract from *Andrographis paniculata* herb 1.0 g Containing andrographolide 10 mg	100 mg	†
Holy Basil *(Ocimum tenuiflorum)* leaf essential oil	10 mg	†

*Percent Daily Values (DV) are based on 2,000 calorie diet.
†Daily Value (DV) not established.

Other Ingredients: Calcium acid phosphate, cellulose, hypromellose, silica, sodium starch glycollate and magnesium stearate.

11. Directions for use: The label should tell you how much and how often the supplement should be taken. For example, "Suggested use: 2-3 tablets daily or as directed."

12. Warnings, cautions and contraindications. For example, MediHerb product labels state: "Not to be used during pregnancy and lactation, unless directed by a health care practitioner. For other contraindications and cautions, consult your health care practitioner. Keep out of reach of children."

Cautions on Herbal Labels

Here are a few "red flags" to look out for:

1. Some manufacturers list herbs with a confusing unit of measure. For example, MediHerb consistently gives the unit of measure of milligrams.

2. Some list a "proprietary" blend which is a list of several herbs, but they don't list the amount of each herb.

3. Some labels have no indication of any active ingredients or quality marker compounds. MediHerb lists these for the product where they are known.

4. Standardized dose is a general term and it can mean anything, so some manufacturers use the word standardized carelessly. MediHerb only uses the term for when the extract is produced to provide consistent levels of marker compounds from batch to batch.

5. Most Herbal products sold over-the-counter are way below therapeutic doses.

6. Some are in Chinese; you have no idea what's in them!

Check Them Out!

How can you decide which herbs to buy? A good rule of thumb is that a liquid herb should taste so strong that you can't taste it straight, while dried herbs should smell as fresh as fresh herbs do. Even capsules should smell and taste like the herb.

MediHerb tablets must legally disintegrate in less than 30 minutes in room temperature water. This means that even in patients with poor digestion MediHerb tablets can quickly and easily be absorbed for best results.

Additionally, a number of MediHerb tablets have a specialized enteric coating which makes the tablets acid resistant. This is important for some herbs which can cause gastric discomfort. Enterically-coated tablets pass through the high acid environment of the stomach safely and then dissolve once they reach the pH neutral environment of the small intestine.

How Do You Know What To Buy?

Obviously, every company is going to try to paint the best picture and encourage you to purchase their herb. Many companies give no indication of how they process herbs. Companies with longstanding reputations, such as Standard Process and MediHerb will have a web site or 1-800 number and places to go for both clinical evidence and information about the company's quality control procedures.

Chapter Seven

Can Herbs Hurt You?

When a client asks, "Can herbs hurt you?" my short answer is, "Only if you choke on them while trying to swallow them, or drop a glass bottle on your toes!"

I can see where some people might shy away from herbs simply because of their names: who wouldn't be cautious about drinking something called Stinging Nettle! For the most part, though, herbs that are properly manufactured (as outlined in this book) and properly taken are safe.

I agree, though, that just because something is "natural," doesn't mean it's safe. So when it comes to herbal safety, we need to look at what has been known as the "traditional" use of herbs. If an herb has a long tradition as being safe and effective, we can have more confidence that it still is safe and effective!

Since herbs have been used for literally thousands of years by so many cultures from around the world, herbalists today have a pretty good idea of which ones are safe and which could be categorized as dangerous.

All over the world, different countries use herbal supplements in place of pharmaceutical drugs. In fact, in many countries, people don't wait until they are sick to go to doctors. Rather, they are trained, as in China, to take herbal remedies as preventative remedies. When they do get sick, they look for herbal supplements. In fact, in some countries, you pay doctors to keep you well, and if you get sick you don't have to pay them. Imagine how this philosophy would change the American healthcare system!

The Safety of Herbs

I've never seen a well documented report that linked taking an specific herb to a death. I like how Kerry Bone puts, it: "If herbs are so dangerous, where are all the dead people?"

Taking into account the general safety of plants, what we have often seen is that in most cases when a person supposedly died because of taking herbs, that person was also, at the same time, taking some type of pharmaceutical drug. The question remains: Was it really the herb that killed them (unlikely) or the drug (very likely).

While herbal remedies have not been subjected to the testing that drugs must undergo to approve their safety, for the most part herbs are safe. However, plants can be potent, and they can interact with prescription drugs.

Some herbs prescribed improperly can cause side effects. I don't know why, but many of my clients like to experiment with herbs. For example, they often have the mentality, "if one is good, more is better." So if I tell them to take one herb a day, they might take two, or three or six! Unfortunately, the "more is better" mentality doesn't work with herbs, especially good herbs such as those manufactured by MediHerb.

A friend of mine told me about a man who took too many of a certain herb to help him sleep. After a day, this man became severely constipated! He got off the herbs and with the help of my friend, was able to sleep and also have good bowel movements (it's the little things in life that matter!).

A Few Cautions About Herbs

People still need to use care when taking herbs. Three potential problems with herbs could be:

*Taking cheap, poorly manufactured herbs

*Taking herbs improperly (too many, or too high of a dose)

*Taking certain herbs with pharmaceutical drugs

How Dangerous Are Herbs?

Recently, I looked up herbs on the internet and I found several pages and links to how dangerous herbs are. When I looked into the discussion, I found, for example, a list of the common herbs listed over and over again, that any reputable herbalist would not even recommend for internal use. (I don't know what I expected; most of the people reporting from these medical web sites are not herbalists!)

What I've noticed is that most medical journal articles focus on the handful of known dangerous herbs and their side effects. One site I saw listed comfrey as linked to liver disease and arnica as causing cardiac toxicity.

Herbalist Christopher Hobbs notes that Comfrey is traditionally used for external purposes to help heal wounds, burns and broken bones, not for internal use. Like Comfrey, Arnica is traditionally used externally, not internally, for strains and inflammation. I've personally used it in my bath water to soothe sore muscles. So it's misleading to call these two herbs "toxic" when they were not designed for internal use, but rather external use only![70]

By the way, Hobbs lists only a handful of potentially toxic herbs: Digitalis, Belladonna, Nux vomica, Aconite, Rauwolfia, and Mandrake, which are not generally sold in stores. Most reputable herbalists only recommend the herbs that are generally recognized as safe. They usually list contraindications as well.[71]

A Few Potentially Toxic Herbs

Herbs that fall between toxic and nontoxic herbs mean that they can be toxic, and are not fatal, but you need to work with a professional, experienced herbalist if you want to use these herbs. They include:

Poke Root, Lobelia, Mistletoe, Chinese Aconite, Bloodroot, Pennyroyal and Germander.[72]

The Scientific "Double Standard"

Mark Blumenthal, Executive Director of the American Botanical Council in Austin, Texas, feels as though herbs have been victimized by a "scientific double standard." When animal studies show some value of herbs, many medical scientists would argue that you can't apply those values to humans. But when an animal suffers harm from any dose of an herb, the same medical scientists call the herb dangerous to humans![73]

Remember, though, that medical journals are generally backed by the drug companies, so wouldn't it be natural for them to point out the dangerous herbs rather than focus on the herbs that are known to replace the drugs they are selling?

Reports of mismedication of Americans hospitalized for adverse reactions to properly prescribed medications make the news for one day and are forgotten. (Remember the drug companies usually fund the media reports.) However, report an herb as harmful and the reports linger on and on and on. Take for example, the herb Kava.

Recently, there were reports of severe liver damage linked to the use of the herb, Kava. However, Kava has had a long history of safe use for depression. Several misleading reports in Europe made health professionals cautious in using Kava. Initially, concern over 29 cases of possible liver damage was reported in Germany and Switzerland. According to Dr. John Lee, what was omitted from the report was that in 21 of these cases, pharmaceutical drugs linked to liver damage were also involved.[74]

Are Herbs Poisonous?

So often people seem to fear taking herbs. I've even asked small children about herbs in my office and they asked, "Aren't they poisonous?" I wondered why they would ask that at such a young age. Where did they hear that? From the drug companies. Herbal critics often call herbs "poisonous."

Rob McCaleb of the National Herb Research Foundation examined reports of the American Association of Poison Control Centers, which collects data on reports of human poisoning. He found that nearly all reports of adverse effects from plants were from consumption of toxic houseplants, not healing herbs. In other words, healing herbs were safe, not poisonous.[75]

Michael Castleman describes an herb that was been discovered in Europe more than 500 years ago, called Noomba. On one hand, it increases alertness, stamina and productivity and on the other hand it can produce insomnia, heartburn, bowel problems and is even linked to heart disease. According to the anthropologists who studied the herb, it's safety was linked to the amount that was consumed.[76]

According to Castleman, Noomba is another name for coffee which he says is probably the most dangerous herb that he even discusses in his book, *The Healing Herbs*. It's the only one he considers addictive and in large amounts, it causes more problems than most others. But it's one of the world's most popular herbs, as we know from the thousands of Starbucks around the country! Most people consider it safe in small amounts.[77]

What About Cancer?

Years ago, scientists discovered that even plant foods contain chemicals that could be dangerous and even cancer causing. Did you know, for example, that one of the best foods known as an anti-cancer agent, the simple carrot, contains arsenic, which is a known poison?

It's possible that if a scientist looks at plant foods under the microscope, most foods could have some type of chemicals in them. But in foods and healing herbs, there are simultaneously cancer preventive-substances, known as antioxidants. It appears that in nature, either healing herbs or plants, there is always safety and balance when the whole plant is in tact.

So, herb critics who focus on finding herbal carcinogens, always find that it's the chemicals that have been isolated (chemically) from the plant that cause cancer. Michael Castleman aptly explains the actions of herb carcinogens are typically offset by the plants' anti-cancer substances. Unless an herb carries a specific warning, healthy people need not fear cancer from ingesting recommended amounts.

Remember years ago when the media reported that taking the supplement beta carotene was dangerous? Yet eating carrots isn't dangerous. The problem was and still is, when people isolate beta carotene and package it as a separate antioxidant. Then it becomes toxic. Beta carotene is one of hundreds of carotonoids, which when taken as a whole food, is not only safe, but protective against cancer.

Reputable herbalists such as Kerry Bone, will tell you that herbs can have side effects, but the majority of herbs used for centuries and used responsibly, are completely safe. In general, healing herbs have far fewer side effects than drugs. However, in each case dosages need to be proper. The more you know about them, the more likely you will have a positive experience of using them safely and effectively.

It is possible, however, that people may experience some types of reactions from taking herbs. Examples of reactions include: stomach upset, nausea, diarrhea, and headache.

Do Herbs Interact With Drugs?

There is a legitimate cause for caution when using herbs, and that is with the use of medications. Here are some tips from herbalist Kerry Bone.

When an herb and drug have similar effects, there is a risk of the effect being excessive if the two treatments are combined without modification of the drug dose. Here are examples of herbs and drugs which work similarly so you don't want to take them simultaneously:[78]

*Ephedra and asthma drugs such as Ventolin

*Aspirin and blood-thinning herbs, such as ginger, tumeric and garlic

*Ginkgo and other blood-thinning herbs with warfarin or aspirin

*Licorice and steroid drugs

*Panax ginseng and MAO inhibitors

*Hawthorn and cardiac glycosides

*Hypotensive herbs and hypotensive drugs

*Herbs which lower blood sugar and insulin or antidiabetic drugs

*St. John's Wort and SSRIs or antidepressants

*Kava and dopamine depleting or antagonist drugs

Two other examples are where the action of the herb counter the desired effect of a drug; for example, don't mix immune enhancing herbs and immunosuppressant drugs.

Other Adverse Interactions

Bone also suggests caution when the herb reinforces an adverse reaction of a drug. Here are potential examples:[79]

*Licorice and thiazide diuretics or diogoxin

*Anthraquinone containing herbs and thiazide diuretics

*Herbs with potential hepatotoxicity, for example, chaparral and hepatotoxic drugs

*Grapefruit juice inhibits the biotransformation of a number of drugs and hence increases their potential for adverse effects.

However, Bone explains that 20% of adverse drug reactions result from drug-drug interactions.

Herb-herb interactions are generally considered to be positive and synergistic. Adverse herb-herb interactions are uncommon.

Bone says that the most common drug involved in herb drug interaction reports is warfarin. In fact, more food and drug interactions have been reported for warfarin than for any other prescription medication.

Bone lists these herbs as possibly interacting with warfarin by increasing its activity:

*Ginkgo

*Garlic

*Dan shen

*Dong quai

*Devil's claw

He lists these herbs that have been reported to possibly decrease the activity of warfarin:[80]

*St. John's wort

*Panax ginseng

Here are some additional tips from herbalist Christopher Hobbs:[81]

*Don't take fiber rich herbs such as psyllium with drugs because it can inhibit absorption of many drugs and also change blood sugar levels.

*Spicy herbs such as cayenne and ginger can enhance absorption of medications.

*Don't mix caffeine-containing herbs like guarana green tea, kola nut, herba matte or chocolate with medications such as Prozac, Zoloft or Paxil.

*Don't take yohimbe if you are on a MAO inhibitor.

If you have a question about herbs, you can also check a reference called the *PDR for Herbal Medicines,* which you can probably order at your local bookstore. Except for taking the wrong amount of an herb, taking certain herbs with certain medications, or taking cheap herbs which may contain toxic chemicals, herbs are safe.

Okay, here it is one more time—the most important thing to do is buy herbs that you know come from a reputable company with high quality assurance standards!

Chapter Eight

How Do You Take Herbs?

Clients frequently ask me about the best way to take herbs. The short answer is to open your mouth and swallow!

But before I discuss how to use herbs appropriately, here is my philosophy on taking herbs.

I tell my clients that their foundation for health is a good diet and regular exercise. I also believe in chiropractic adjustments and have found that some people absolutely need to address their spinal issues before they can truly have great health. We refer clients to chiropractors quite often.

I'm also an advocate of taking whole-food nutritional supplements and the ones I use are from Standard Process. (For more information on whole-food supplements for health, see the list of the books I have written at the end of this book.)

Since Standard Process supplements are food, they help make up for nutritional deficiencies fairly quickly and rarely cause any side effects. For example, a client named Karen tested low on the B complex. I recommended that she take Standard Process Cataplex B®, a whole food B complex. She also needed a multiple vitamin, for which I recommended Standard Process Catalyn.® And she was low in magnesium, for which I recommended Magnesium Lactate. Most of my clients need a minimum of three or four nutritional Standard Process supplements. Standard Process products and MediHerb products combine well. So I recommend herbal products as they seem appropriate. For example, Karen told me she had various cravings, so I added Cataplex GTF® which helped with the sugar cravings.

Later, I added the MediHerb, Gymnema to her protocol which supported her blood sugar levels and reduced carbohydrate cravings as well.

General Tips for Taking Herbs

1. Some people take too many herbs. Use only the recommended amounts and use them only for the recommended amount of time. Make sure the herb you are taking is appropriate for the condition you have. When in doubt, follow the suggested amount that is already written on the label.

If you are elderly, or someone sensitive to drugs and supplements, start with very low doses.

2. Use the right herb and part of the plant. Read the label and look for possible contraindications and better still, see a qualified natural healthcare professional. It's best if you purchase your herbs from a reputable company, and use them under the care of a person trained in herbology.

3. If you are taking medications, work with a health professional, even though most herbs are safe. Some herbs interact with drugs and others don't. At the very least, take your herbs and medications at different times of the day.

(MediHerb can supply your healthcare professional with a chart of the Contraindications and Cautions for MediHerb Botanicals. See page 103 on how to herbal find products and a natural healthcare professional.)

Use herbal products for minor conditions, not when there is a life threatening situation.

4. Stop taking an herb if you have any unusual reactions. Try a few days later, and if you still have an allergic reaction, discontinue the herb. As I mentioned in the previous chapter, examples of reactions include: stomach upset, nausea, diarrhea, and headache.

Most herbs are extremely safe when taken properly. Sometimes a mild allergy type reaction might occur because the herb quality is poor, because the combination of herbs are not compatible, or because it was contaminated either in the growing or manufacturing process. Take the right dose. Anything taken in excess can cause side effects. Again, be sure to buy herbs from a reputable source.

5. Don't take herbs if you are pregnant, trying to get pregnant or lactating. Herbs that are safe for adults may not be safe for the unborn. Don't give herbs to children under the age of two, unless with the guidance of a qualified herbalist. Be conservative on dosing for children; it's best to work with a health professional when working with children.

6. I encourage you to try to take your herbal supplements three times a day with your meals. If you can't take them with meals, then take them before or after you eat. If you can't manage to take them three times, then cut the dosage in half and take them twice a day. Just get them in every day!

It's always necessary to follow a healthy diet when you use medicinal herbs since they supplement the diet; they don't replace good eating habits. You are probably familiar with the guidelines: Don't eat white flour, white sugar, soda, coffee, tea, processed foods and fried foods. (For some people, this was their entire diet!)

Keep your herbs tightly capped in a cool place and they should last two to three years. Check the expiration date which is found on the tablet (See page 80).

How Long Do You Take Them?

Most clients ask me, "Am I supposed to take herbs every day for the rest of my life?" With therapeutic herbs, it all depends on what you need the herbal therapy for. A good rule of thumb is to take them one month for every year that you have had the condition. However, people with chronically low immune function may want to take herbs indefinitely.

Some herbs, such as garlic, mint or cayenne are wonderful spices that can be eaten daily forever!

Dosing for Children

Clients frequently ask me about how to give children herbs or supplements. Here are suggestions for children who can swallow tablets:

Ages 12 and older take the adult dose

Ages 6-12 take half the adult dose

Ages 6 and under take one fourth the adult dose

For children who can't swallow tablets, here's an idea. Take liquid formulas or grind up the tablets in a coffee grinder and add the powder to a protein drink, applesauce, or some other food that the child will eat.

Types of Herbal Products

There are several ways to take herbs, including in teas, infusions, tinctures, vinegars, powders and so on. Below I list the most common ways herbs are sold.

Tablets are made from pressing herbs with a binder. Tablets can often be coated which makes them easier to swallow.

Liquid Extracts are considered to be one of the best ways to take herbs since the active ingredients are more concentrated.

Capsules are easy to swallow and don't generally contain binders or fillers. Capsules can contain the powders of leaves, roots or extracts from herbs.

Benefits of Liquid Herbals

Liquid herbals can be customized to each client. Your natural health professional who has the license to sell MediHerb liquid herbals can combine liquid herbs together. Here are some advantages for using liquids:

1. They are easier to take. Since the herbal protocols are combined, the client only has to pour out of one bottle, not four or five.

2. Liquids are a great way to get a potent dose in a concentrated form, so they are cost effective.

3. Liquids are great for children and adults who have difficulty swallowing tablets. These are also helpful for the elderly, or people with poor digestion.

4. Herbal extracts are readily absorbed, so the active constituents can be delivered much faster than the majority of tablets or capsules which must first be broken down by the digestive tract. This is especially helpful for people with slow digestion or for those who need immediate results.

The downside is the strong herbal taste and the alcohol content which is often used. Taste issues can be overcome by adding the herbs to red grape juice.

Alcohol liquid extracts are not recommended for people with liver problems; find herbs made without alcohol.

Teas are easy to use and the cheapest way to take herbs. There are many delicious blends of herbal teas on the market, but they are not recommended as the primary way of using herbs therapeutically.

You'll also find lozenges available, often used for fighting a cold or allergies. Look for the ones without refined white sugar. Additionally, ointments, creams and salves are helpful ways to treat rashes or skin wounds.

Sometimes herbs, like Ginkgo, for example, are added to your cereal or potato chips in an attempt to make them more marketable. It's unlikely that you will get enough herbs to have any effect, but you might learn something about herbs by reading the label on the boxes!

Part Three of this book lists some of the more popular MediHerb products, a few herbal recipes, and some information on how to find herbs and a natural health professional.

In closing, I pray for God's blessings on your journey to great health.

PART THREE

Herbs for Life

Chapter Nine

Popular MediHerb Products for Great Health

In this chapter, I'll highlight the most popular MediHerb liquids and tablets that I use in my practice. (See their site, www.MediHerb.com for information on them.)

MediHerb Single Liquid Extracts

Aloe Vera Soothes inflammation of the gastrointestinal tract and is a great food for digestive problems.

Astragalus Strengthens the immune system, supports the adrenal glands and provides energy.

Bacopa A tonic for memory and cognitive functions such as Attention Deficit Disorder.

Bilberry Prevents night blindness and cataracts; supports eye health as an antioxidant.

Black Cohosh Relieves hot flashes and menstrual cramps.

Cat's Claw Internal blood cleanser which helps to prevent tumors and build the immune system; it's also an anti-inflammatory herb.

Chamomile Good for indigestion and has a calming effect.

Chaste Tree Especially helpful for symptoms of PMS, balances the menstrual cycle and promotes fertility.

Cranberry Helps prevent bladder infection and urinary tract infections by reducing the ability of bacteria to adhere to the bladder wall.

Dandelion Helps increase the production of bile and has a positive effect on liver detoxification pathways; it's a diuretic and liver tonic.

Don Quai Promotes healthy female reproductive system function and eases the pain of normal menstruation.

Echinacea Premium Combines the roots of the Echinacea angustifolia and the Echinacea purpurea to enlist properties unique to each. It helps boost immune system and white blood cell production; it's great for colds and flu.

Eleuthero (Ginseng, Siberian) Used to help a person adapt to stress; especially for chronic fatigue; it restores and enhances immune system function, and acts as a general tonic.

Feverfew Promotes the body's normal resistance function, and encourages healthy circulation so it helps relieve headaches, especially migraines.

Ganoderma & Shitake The combination of these unique mushrooms can help to stimulate healthy immune response, and encourage adaptive response to occasional everyday stress.

Garlic Helps lower cholesterol and supports heart health; it also supports immune function, and helps fight yeast infections.

Ginkgo Biloba Improves oxygen and circulation to the brain; it helps memory loss and supports brain health.

Globe Artichoke Stimulates bile flow and production, so it's helpful due to its natural cholesterol lowering effect; it also helps restore the liver.

Golden Seal helps maintain healthy mucous membranes; it assists in maintaining healthy breathing passages to support free and clear breathing, and it helps maintain healthy mucous function.

Gota Kola Improves circulation in the veins and stimulates healing.

Gymnema Maintains healthy blood-sugar levels when combined with a balanced diet and it helps maintain normal cholesterol levels.

Hawthorn An all around general heart support herb which is helpful for lowering blood pressure, and preventing angina pectoris and a weak or enlarged heart.

Licorice An adrenal tonic which also helps as an anti-inflammatory and protects the stomach lining.

Milk Thistle (Silymarin) Helps the liver not absorb toxins; it's an antioxidant, and supports liver regeneration.

Pau D'arco Anti-microbial and anti-tumor, it's also an immune stimulating herb.

St. John's Wort Clinically proven to help mild to moderate depression; also shown to be effective against enveloped viruses, which includes measles, mumps, herpes, hepatitis B and C, and cytomegalovirus.

Saw Palmetto Has been shown to work as well as prescription medicine for benign enlarged prostate with no side effects.

Tribulus Used for debilitating states of sexual organs and impotence.

Uva Ursi Used as a diuretic and urinary antiseptic.

Valerian An overall tonic to relax muscles and reduce anxiety; it's helpful for sleep problems.

MediHerb Complex Tablet Formulas

Albizia Complex A combination of Albizia, Baical Skullcap and Feverfew. This combination helps maintain normal upper respiratory tract and skin function and helps alleviate allergies.

Andrographis Complex A combination of Echinacea, Holy Basil and Andrographis to enhance immune system and support respiratory system functions.

Bacopa Complex Combines Schisandra, Eleuthero root, Bacopa and Rosemary oil to enhance mental clarity, support cognitive function and nourish the nervous system.

Bilberry Supports vascular integrity, connective tissue; it also supports healthy eyes and provides antioxidant protection.

Boswellia Complex contains four herbs used for all inflammatory conditions such as arthritis, bursitis, rheumatism, fibromyalgia, Crohn's disease and ulcerative colitis.

Broncafect® Contains Licorice root, Pleurisy root, Echinacea purpurea root, White Horehound herb, Ginger and Thyme oil. It supports healthy respiratory tract function, throat tissue and mucus flow. It's especially good for acute infections.

Burdock Complex Contains Burdock, Sheep Sorrel, Slippery Elm, Rhubarb. It enhances immune response, supports the body's organs of elimination and maintains healthy blood and skin.

Colax The combination of Dill Seed, Cascara, Yellow Dock, Dandelion Root and Chamomile help support healthy bowel function, cleanse the lower digestive tract, and relieve mild constipation.

Cramplex Contains Cramp Bark, Corydalis, Ginger, Raspberry Leaf and Wild Yam. This combination of herbs which can help ease occasional spasms of smooth muscle including those associated with the menstrual cycle; it provides relief from discomfort associated with menstruation.

DermaCo® Contains Sarsaparilla, Cleavers, Oregon Grape, Burdock and Yellow Dock. This combination helps encourage the healthy function of the organs of elimination, promotes normal healthy skin renewal and integrity, maintains healthy skin, and cleanses the blood.

DiGest® Contains Gentian, Milk Thistle, Ginger, Dandelion Root, Tangerine and Chamomile oil which help stimulate appetite, and support healthy digestion and intestinal function.

Eleuthero (Siberian Ginseng) Is used to help a person adapt to stress; especially for chronic fatigue; it restores and enhances immune system function, and acts as a general tonic.

Euphrasia Complex® Combines the herbs Eyebright, Golden Rod, Echinacea purpurea root, Golden Seal and Cayenne. These help maintain healthy and normal mucous secretion in the sinuses and nasal passages and assist in maintaining healthy breathing passages to support free and clear breathing.

Evening Primrose Oil Contains essential fatty acids of the omega-6 series which promote healthy skin, and ease discomfort associated with the menstrual cycle and premenstrual syndrome.

Horsechestnut Complex Contains Butcher's Broom root, Horsechestnut seed, and Ginkgo biloba. It supports circulation, venous integrity, varicose veins, inflammation.

Livco® Contains Schisandra, Rosemary and MilkThistle which support liver detoxification and elimination of toxins.

Livton® Complex Contains Globe Artichoke, Dandelion, Milk Thistle, Greater Celandine, and Fringe Tree root bark. This combination supports healthy liver and gallbladder function, and promotes bile flow.

Nevaton® Contains Schisandra, Damiana, Skullcap, and St. John's Wort. Great for relaxing the nervous system, for mood swings and stress.

PulmaCo® Contains Malabar Nut Tree, Chinese Skullcap, Turmeric, Ginkgo, Grindelia and Fennel oil and helps assist in maintaining healthy breathing passages to support free and clear breathing; it supports the body's natural ability to break up and expel respiratory secretions.

ResCo® Contains Licorice, Mullein, Euphorbia, Grindelia, Ginger, Fennel and Thyme. It supports mucous membranes, promotes healthy airway passages respiratory function and resistance. It's especially good for chronic conditions.

Saligesic White Willow stem bark. It's commonly used to replace aspirin for fever, pain and inflammation.

Serenoa Complex Helps to support healthy urinary tract and prostate gland function and to facilitate proper urine flow.

Thyroid Complex® Contains Bladderwack, Withania and Bacopa. It's an excellent support for the thyroid.

Vitanox® Contains Rosemary, Green Tea, Turmeric and Grape Seed which provide strong antioxidant protection and support healthy circulation and vascular integrity.

Wild Yam Complex Contains Wild Yam, False Unicorn, Sage, Korean Ginseng and St. John's Wort. It provides relief from discomfort associated with menopause.

Withania Complex Contains Licorice, Withania (Ashwaganda), Skullcap, Korean Ginseng. An adrenal and general tonic, it's especially great for chronic fatigue.

Wormwood Contains Stemona root, Black Walnut green hulls, and Wormwood. It's effective for eliminating intestinal parasites.

Chapter Ten

Handy Herbal Recipes

The following recipes are from Kerry Bone and used with his permission. They are all specifically made with MediHerb products. No guarantee can be made if you make these without MediHerbal liquid products.

Feminine Douche

2 cups warm water (or Calendula tea)
1 tablespoon apple cider vinegar
2 drops Tea Tree oil
5 mL Oregon Grape 1:2
5 mL Pau d'Arco
3 mL Echinacea Premium 1:2
Mix together and douche using a very slow, gentle flow.

Herbal Face Mask

4 tablespoons (3 oz) oatmeal
Warm water
1 clove garlic, crushed
5 mL Calendula 1:2
50 mL Golden Seal 1:3
Add enough warm water to the oatmeal to form a stiff paste. Add Calendula, Golden Seal and freshly crushed garlic. Apply mask to face and leave for approximately 3-5 minutes only (fresh garlic in contact with the skin can burn if left for long periods of time.) Be careful to avoid contact with the eyes. Rinse with warm water and follow with the Herbal Face Wash. Use this mask once per week to promote normal healthy skin.

(Caution: Do not use in known cases of contact dermatitis or allergy to garlic.)

Herbal Face Wash

50 mL Calendula 1:2
50 mL Echinacea Premium 1:2

Add 2 ½ mL of herbal mixture to approximately 100 mL warm water and bathe face. Pat face dry with a soft cotton towel. Use this herbal face wash 2-3 times per day to promote normal healthy skin.

Mouthwash

½ cup of water (or peppermint tea for flavor)
3 mL Oregon Grape 1:2
3 mL Sage 1:2
3 mL Echinacea Premium Blend 1:2

Mix ingredients together, swish and swallow three times a day, after meals.

Soothing Eyebath

8 drops Eyebright 1:2
8 drops Chamomile High Grade 1:2

(Caution if allergy to the daisy family)

Put herbs in heat resistant container. Pour ½ cup of boiling water over this mixture to dissipate the alcohol. Allow to cool and fill eyebath cup. This will be enough mixture to fill four, 1 oz. eyebath cups. Use fresh solution for each eye. Use within 4 hours. If a stronger solution is needed, use 8 drops of Golden Seal (1:3) instead of Chamomile.

Saline Nasal Spray

Base
30 mL purified water
¼ teaspoon sea salt
5 mL glycerin
Mix together.

Add herbs
1 mL Albizia 1:2
1 mL Baical Skullcap 1:2
2 mL Eyebright 1:2
2 mL Golden Seal 1:3

Mix base and herbs together and pour into a clean, empty saline nasal spray bottle. Spray into each nostril as needed. (Contraindicated in infection or blockage of the sinuses.) (Caution: potential allergic reaction could occur with use in each of these recipes. If you have any difficulty, please discontinue and consult your health professional.)

Chapter Eleven

How to Find Herbs and Natural Health Professionals

In writing this book on herbal supplements, one of my goals was to help the reader understand the importance of herbs for both preventing disease and healing.

You wouldn't eat junk food while trying to improve your health, and you certainly wouldn't want to use "junk" vitamins (synthetic or crystalline extract vitamins), that are often sold in stores. In my book, *Why Do I Need Whole-Food Supplements*, I have explained with clinical research why whole-food vitamin supplements are the only type of supplements that promote healing. Standard Process Inc. sells whole-food vitamin supplements through natural health professionals. They also distribute products made by MediHerb, the cold-processed, professional herbal company that I have referred to throughout this book. These herbs are some of the best on the market in the world.

Today's herbalists, such as Kerry Bone, respect time honored tradition and look to research about the properties of the whole plant rather than isolated properties. Herbalists such as Bone believe that the power of herbal medicine lies in the synergy of all of the plant's ingredients or components. (I like to refer to him as the herbal Royal Lee! But I think others call him Mr. Echinacea, after his love for the herb.)

So when you are ready to start using herbs and/or seek professional help to improve any health concern you have, it will be important for you to find a "natural" health professional who can provide the products I have recommended in this book. The types of "natural" health professionals you want to assist you in getting well are Naturopathic Doctors (N.D.), Clinical Nutritionists (C.N.), Certified Clinical Nutritionists (C.C.N.), and any doctor (D.C., M.D., D.D., D.O., D.D.S., Ph.D.) or pharmacist who has studied and completed post-graduate studies in Clinical Nutrition. Health Professionals who wish to take a certification course in herbology can go to the website www.herbaleducation.com.au for information about the Australian College of Phytotherapy.

About Standard Process/MediHerb Products

Standard Process and MediHerb products are only available through "natural" health professionals as listed above. If you purchase herbs or vitamins from a health food store or through the mail, I can't guarantee you the same results as with a clinical product such as Standard Process or MediHerb.

For more information on Standard Process or MediHerb, talk to the professional who gave you this book or call 1-800-848-5061 to find a healthcare professional in your area.

Standard Process Inc. and MediHerb
1200 West Royal Lee Drive
Palmyra, WI 53156-0904
1-800-848-5061

If you would like to contact me, my address is listed below. My bio and booklist are at the end of this book.

Lorrie Medford, CN
Life Design Nutrition
9726 E. 42nd St. Suite 231
Tulsa, OK 74146
918-664-4483
918-664-0300 (fax)
Web address: lifedesignnutrition.com
E-mail: Lorrie@lifedesignnutrition.com

Endnotes

1. Earl L. Mindell, R.Ph, PhD and Virginia Hopkins, M.A. *Prescription Alternatives*, 2nd edition. (Los Angeles, CA: Keats Publishing, 1999), p. 87.

2. Cancer Facts and Figures, 2003, American Cancer Society. www.cancer.gov.

3. World Health Organization Statistical Information (Web address: www.who.int/home-page)

4. See the website for the Surgeon General Report www.surgeon general.gov/topics/obesity/calltoaction/toc.htm - 4k - Jul 29, 2004.

5. World Health Organization Statistical Information (Web address: www.who.int/home-page)

6. Patrick Quillin, Ph.D. *Beating Cancer With Nutrition* (Tulsa, OK: The Nutrition Times Press, Inc., 2001), p. 23.

7. Lorrie Medford, C.N. *Why Do I Feel So Lousy?* (Tulsa, OK: LDN Publishing, 2003), pp.29-33.

8. Anderson and Jensen *Empty Harvest* (Garden City Park, NY: Avery Publishers), 1990, p. 37.

9. Anderson and Jensen, pp. 39-40.

10. Dr. John Lee Medical Letter, September 2003, p. 4.

11. Peter Jennings, ABC News, December 2003, "How To Get Fat Without Really Trying."

12. Paul A. Stitt *Beating the Food Giants* (Manitowoc, WI: Natural Press, 1995), p. 117.

13. Stitt p. 117-118.

14. Marion Nestle *Food Politics* (Berkeley, CA: University of California Press, 2002), p. 22.

15. Nestle, p. 179.

16. Marian Burros, "Additives in Advice on Food?" *New York Times,* Nov. 15, 1995, Vol. 145, p. C1.

17. Burros, p. C1.

18. Anderson and Jensen, pp. 39-40.

19. World Health Organization Statistical Information (Web address: www.who.int/home-page)

20. Jethro Kloss *Back to Eden: The Classic Guide to Herbal Medicine, Natural Foods and Home Remedies Since 1939* (Twin Lakes, WI: Lotus Press, 1939), p. 47.

21. Kloss, p. 48.

22. Kloss, p. 51.

23. Kerry Bone and Simon Mills *The Principles and Practice of Phytotherapy Modern Herbal Medicine* (London, England: Churchill Livingstone, 2000), p. 4.

24. Michael Castleman *The Healing Herbs: The Ultimate Guide to the Creative Power of Nature's Medicines* (New York, New York: Bantam Books, 1995), p. 19.

25. Castleman, p. 19.

26. Bone and Mills, p. 12.

27. Bone and Mills, p. 12.

28. Castleman, p. 21.

29. Bone and Mills, p. 13.

30. Bone and Mills, p. 23.

31. Castleman, p. 23.

32. Kloss, p. 58.

33. Bone and Mills, p. 13.

34. Bone and Mills, p. 14.

35. Art Ulene, M.D. Dr. *Art Ulene's Complete Guide to Vitamins, Minerals and Herbs* (New York, New York: Avery Books, 2004), p. 20.

36. Louise Tenney, MH *Today's Herbal Health* (Pleasant Grove, Utah: Woodland Publishing, 2000), p. 11.

37. Phyllis A. Balch, CNC and James F. Balch, M.D. *Prescription for Nutritional Healing,* 3rd edition (New York, New York: Avery Books, 2000), pp. 85-88.

38. Lorna Vanderhaeghe and Patrick J.D. Bouic, Ph.D. *The Immune System Cure* (New York, NY: Kensington Books, 1999), p. 5.

39. The Burton Goldberg Group *Alternative Medicine: The Definitive Guide* (Fife, Washington: Future Medicine Publishing, Inc.,1995), p. 253.

40. World Health Organization Statistical Information (Web address: www.who.int/home-page)

41. Dr. Royal Lee, "How and Why Synthetic Poisons Are Being Sold as Imitations of Natural Foods and Drugs," December 1948.

42. Tenney, *Today's Herbal Health,* p. 11.

43. Mark Pedersen *Nutritional Herbology: A Reference Guide to Herbs* (Warsaw, IN: Wendell W. Whitman Company, 1994), p. 5.

44. Pedersen, p. 5.

45. Earl Mindell, R.Ph., Ph.D. *Earl Mindell's New Herb Bible* (New York, New York, Fire Side Books, 2000), p. 13.

46. Louise Tenney, *Louise Tenney's Nutritional Guide With Food Combining* (Pleasant Grove, UT: Woodland Publishing, Inc., 1994), p. 47.

47. Tenney, *Louise Tenney's Nutritional Guide With Food Combining*, p. 47.

48. Janet Zand, LAC. OMD, Allan N. Spreen, MD, CNC, James B. LaValle, RPh, M.D. *Smart Medicine for Healthier Living* (Garden City Park, New York: Avery Publishing Group, 1999), p. 23.

49. Pedersen, p. 5.

50. Balch, p. 5.

51. Balch, p. 3.

52. Christopher Hobbs, *Herbal Remedies for Dummies* (New York, NY: Wiley Publishing, 1998), p. 11.

53. Rick Weiss, "Correctly Prescribed Drugs Take Heavy Toll," *The Washington Post,* April 15, 1998.

54. Dr. John Lee Medical Letter, March 2002, p. 3.

55. Dr. Marcus Laux, "Breakthrough Therapies for Detecting and Preventing Heart Disease," p. 4.

56. Dr. Bruce West, *Health Alert,* Monterey, CA: 2001, Volume 18, Issue 6, pp. 1-2.

57. Earl L. Mindell, R.Ph, PhD and Virginia Hopkins, M.A. *Prescription Alternatives*, 2nd edition. (Los Angeles, CA: Keats Publishing, 1999), p. vii-ix.

58. Dr. Bruce West, *Health Alert,* Vol. 19, Issue 3, p. 8.

59. Dr. Bruce West, *Health Alert,* Vol. 19, Issue 1, p. 6.

60. Dr. Bruce West, *Health Alert,* July 2004, Volume 21, Issue 7,. p.4.

61. Dr. Marcus Laux, *Naturally Well Today Newsletter,* February 2004, p. 1.

62. Donna Gates *The Stevia Story* (Atlanta, GA: BED Publications, 1997), p. 29.

63. Web site Stevia.com.

64. *Alternative Medicine Magazine,* July/Aug 2004, p. 96.

65. Bone and Mills, p. 108.

66. Bone and Mills, p. 109.

67. Bone and Mills, p. l09.

68. Kerry Bone, *Definitive Course in Practical Herbal Therapy,* Module One, Quality and Safety Issues in Herbal Medicine.

69. Art Ulene, p. 22.

70. Hobbs, p. 22.

71. Hobbs, p. 24.

72. Hobbs, p. 27-29.

73. Castlemen, p. 33.

74. John Lee, M.D., *Medical Letter,* July 2001, p. 2.39.

75. Hobbs, p. 21.

76. Castleman, p. 31.

77. Castleman, pp. 31-32.

78. Kerry Bone Herbal Seminar

79. Kerry Bone Herbal Seminar

80. Kerry Bone, Herbal Seminar

81. Hobbs, pp. 22-24.

I have made every effort possible to check the accuracy of material quoted. If there is any question, or a possible mistake in quoting of any material, necessary changes will be made in future printings.

Index

Order Form

Please Print

Name _____

Address _____

City _____ State _____ Zip _____

Phone _____

E-mail _____

METHOD OF PAYMENT

Check _____ Credit Card: Visa_____ Mastercard_____

Card number _____ Exp. date_____

Authorization Signature _____

ITEM	QTY	PRICE
Why Can't I Lose Weight? ($17.95)		
Why Can't I Lose Weight Cookbook ($17.95)		
Why Can't I Stay Motivated? ($14.95)		
Why Am I So Grumpy, Dopey and Sleepy? ($11.95)		
Why Am I So Wacky? ($11.95)		
Why Eat Like Jesus Ate? ($11.95)		
Why Do I Need Whole Food Supplements? ($9.95)		
Why Do I Feel So Lousy? ($9.95)		
Why Do I Really Need Herbs? ($9.95)		
Subtotal		
Shipping & Handling Add 15%		
(Add 8% if resident of OK) Tax		
Total		

Send check or money order to:

Life Design Nutrition

Lorrie Medford, CN

PO Box 54007

Tulsa, OK 74155

918-664-4483

918-664-0300 (fax)

E-mail orders: lorrie@lifedesignnutrition.com

www.lifedesignnutrition.com